METABOLIC DISEASES - LABORATORY AND CLINICAL RESEARCH

# LYSOSOMAL STORAGE DISEASES

## PATHOBIOLOGY AND THERAPEUTIC CONSIDERATIONS

# METABOLIC DISEASES - LABORATORY AND CLINICAL RESEARCH

Additional books in this series can be found on Nova's website under the Series tab.

Additional e-books in this series can be found on Nova's website under the e-book tab.

METABOLIC DISEASES - LABORATORY AND CLINICAL RESEARCH

# LYSOSOMAL STORAGE DISEASES

## PATHOBIOLOGY AND THERAPEUTIC CONSIDERATIONS

GREGORY M. PASTORES

NOVA BIOMEDICAL

*New York*

**Library of Congress Cataloging-in-Publication Data**

ISBN: 978-1-63484-661-5

*Published by Nova Science Publishers, Inc. † New York*

# Contents

# Preface

> *The optimism of science is two-fold: that its methods might reveal, one tiny pixel at a time, more of the wonder of the natural world, and that this knowledge might be able to solve practical human problems. There is abundant evidence in both cases that this optimism is justified.*
>
> Georgina Ferry (2009)

Since the publication of an earlier monograph, entitled *Lysosomal storage disorders (LSD): Principles and Practice* (World Scientific Publishing Company, Singapore, 2010), there have been significant advances in knowledge regarding the pathobiology of the lysosome. In parallel, major developments have also ensued on the therapeutic front. However, there remain major gaps. For instance, there is incomplete understanding of mechanistic links between the accumulating substrate and disease mechanisms that ultimately mediate cellular dysfunction and death. Moreover, although there are several disease-modifying treatments, for the majority of symptomatic patients the benefit appears modest, especially when viewed in terms of cost and life-long commitment to intravenous infusions (in the case of enzyme therapy). Furthermore, none of the currently available treatments have a major impact on the central nervous system-related aspects of the phenotype. The multiplicity of putative disease pathways suggests combination therapy ultimately may be required to achieve an optimal outcome. In any event, early diagnosis appears critical as residual disease can be a continuing burden for treated patients, limiting physical and functional well-being.

In the current publication, the aim will be to summarize the latest findings regarding the consequences of lysosomal dysfunction, which occur primarily because of a disruption in the sequential degradation of various substrates generated by cellular turnover. Prior to delving into deleterious cellular events, the nature and physiology of the lysosome will be reviewed.

Several mechanisms of disease have been described; although seemingly discrete and initially involving different subcellular compartments (e.g., autophagosome and the lysosome), these events are interconnected. Moreover, even when a particular defect is identified (e.g., impairment of mitophagy), the observed changes may be mediated by distinctive processes; which calls attention to myriad ways cells can respond to injury. In each of the relevant sections, disease-specific observations are described.

Although there are indications of shared disease pathways, given the variety of substrates involved, differences in underlying etiology and heterogeneity in disease expression (i.e., age at onset, rate of disease progression, and the presence of central nervous system involvement with certain clinical subtypes), it is anticipated there will be aspects particular to a given condition. Indeed, one of the challenges in understanding the pathophysiology of individual LSDs lies in determination of which pathologic features play a dominant role. It should be noted, the majority of observations relating to pathophysiology have been derived from investigations of animal models, primarily mice subjected to genetic manipulation. Although of great interest, especially in relation to changes that are evident prior to the onset of symptoms, the relevance to human subjects of certain findings made in animal models remains to be confirmed. Regarding investigations that have involved human tissues, primarily cultured fibroblasts, there is uncertainty regarding the generalizability of findings to different cells types, especially neurons.

Aspects relating to clinical presentation, diagnostic confirmation and assessment of disease severity were covered in detail in *LSD: Principles and Practice.* An approach to patients suspected of having LSD, proceeding from the chief complaint, is shown in Figure 1.

Topics covered in the book are grouped into three sections: (1) physiologic events involving or occurring within the confines of the lysosome; (2) cellular perturbations implicated in lysosomal storage disease; and (3) therapeutic strategies and views relating to genetic screening and counselling. Background material and additional information are provided in boxed sections at the end of each chapter. Diagrams are included to facilitate greater understanding of relevant themes. The subject matters that are discussed can be found scattered over several publications; the current monograph attempts to collate several perspectives into a coherent narrative and serve as a convenient resource.

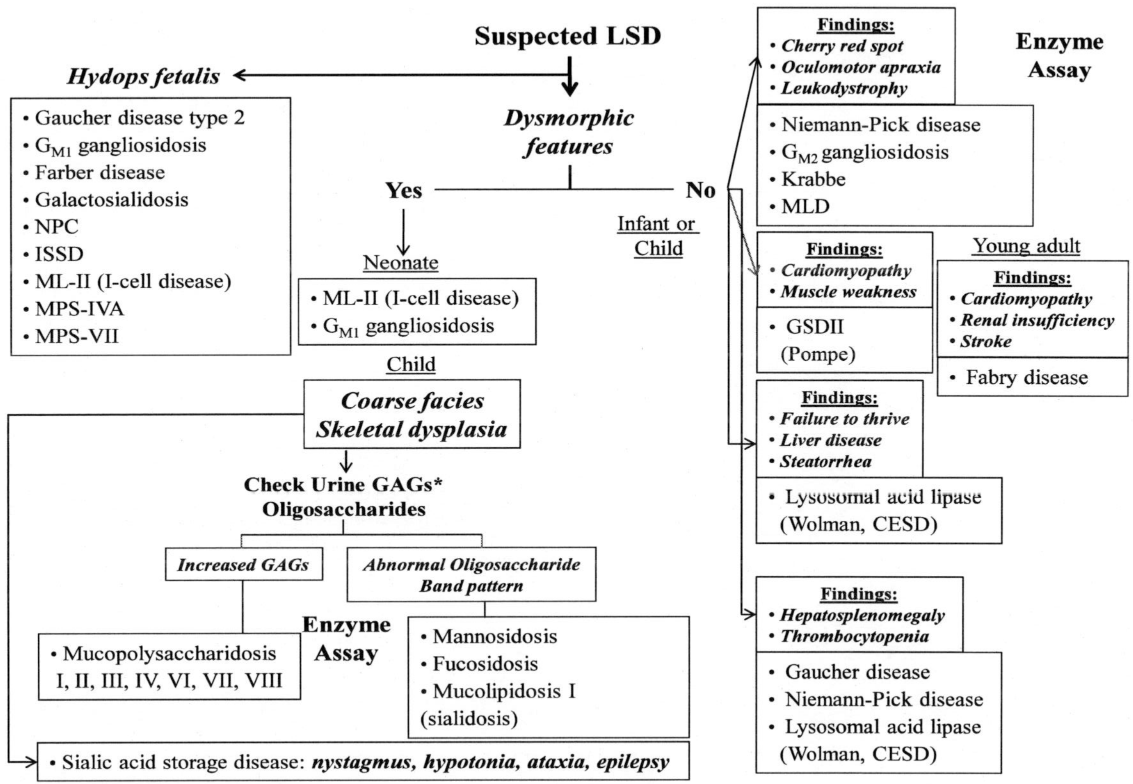


Figure 1. Differential diagnosis.

**Table 1. Lysosomal storage disorders, classified according to the primary storage material**

| **Stored Substrate** | **Disease** | **Enzyme/Protein Deficiency** | **Gene Locus** |
|---|---|---|---|
| SPHINGOLIPIDS | | | |
| $GM_2$ gangliosides, glycolipids, globoside oligosaccharides | Tay–Sachs disease | α Subunit of β-hexosaminidase | *HEXA,* 15q23 |
| | $GM_2$ gangliosidosis (three types) | | |
| | Sandhoff disease | β Subunit of β-hexosaminidase | *HEXB,* 5q13.3 |
| | $GM_2$ gangliosidosis | | |
| | $GM_2$ gangliosidosis, AB variant | $GM_2$ activator | *GM2A,* 5q33.1 |
| $GM_1$ gangliosides, oligosaccharides, keratan sulfate, glycolipids | $GM_1$ gangliosidosis (three types) | β-D-Galactosidase | *GLB1,* 3p22.3 |
| Sulfatides | Metachromatic leukodystrophy | Arylsulfatase A (galactose-3-sulfatase) | *ARSA,* 22q13.33 |
| $GM_1$ gangliosides, sphingomyelin, glycolipids, sulfatide | Metachromatic leukodystrophy variant | Saposin B activator | *PSAP,* 10q22.1 |
| Galactosylceramides | Krabbe disease | Galactocerebrosidase | *GALC,* 14q31.3 |
| α-Galactosylsphingolipids, oligosaccharides | Fabry disease | α-Galactosidase A | *GLA,* Xq22.1 |
| Glucosylceramide, globosides | Gaucher disease (three types) | β-Glucosidase | *GBA,* 1q22 |
| Glucosylceramide, globosides | Gaucher disease (variant) | Saposin C | *PSAP,* 10q22 |
| Ceramide | Farber disease (seven types) | Acid ceramidase | *ASAH1,* 8p22 |
| Sphingomyelin | Niemann–Pick disease types A and B | Sphingomyelinase | *SMPD1,* 11p15.4 |

| **Stored Substrate** | **Disease** | **Enzyme/Protein Deficiency** | **Gene Locus** |
|---|---|---|---|
| MUCOPOLYSACCHARIDES (GLYCOSAMINOGLYCANS) | | | |
| Dermatan sulfate and heparan sulfate | MPS I, Hurler–Scheie | α-L-Iduronidase | *IDUA,* 4p16.3 |
| | MPS II, Hunter | Iduronate-2-sulfatase | *IDS,* Xq28 |
| Heparan sulfate | MPS IIIA, Sanfilippo A | Sulfamidase | *SGSH,* 17q25.3 |
| | MPS IIIB, Sanfilippo B | α-*N*-Acetylglucosaminidase | *NAGLU,* 17q21.2 |
| | MPS IIIC, Sanfilippo C | Acetyl-CoA: α-glucosaminide-*N*-acetyltransferase | *HGSNAT,* 8p11.21 |
| | MPS IIID, Sanfilippo D | *N*-Acetylglucosamine-6-sulfatase | *GNS,* 12q14.3 |
| Keratan sulfate | MPS IVA, Morquio A | Galactosamine-6-sulfatase | *GALNS,* 16q24.3 |
| | MPS IVB, Morquio B | β-D-Galactosidase | *GLB1,* 3p22.3 |
| Dermatan sulfate | MPS VI, Maroteaux–Lamy | *N*-Acetylgalactosamine-4-sulfatase | *ARSB,* 5q13–14 |
| Dermatan sulfate and heparan sulfate | MPS VII, Sly | β-D-Glucuronidase | *GUSB,* 7q11.21 |
| Hyaluronan | MPS IX, Natowicz | Hyaluronoglucosaminidase | *HYAL1,* 3p21.31 |
| GLYCOGEN | | | |
| Glycogen | Pompe disease, glycogen storage disease type IIA | Acid α-D-Glucosidase | *GAA,* 17q25.3 |
| Glycogen | Danon disease | Lysosomal associated membrane protein-2 (LAMP-2) | *LAMP2,* Xq24 |
| OLIGOSACCHARIDES/GLYCOPEPTIDES | | | |
| α-Mannoside | α-Mannosidosis | α-Mannosidase | *MAN2B1,* 19p13.2 |
| β-Mannoside | β-Mannosidosis | β-Mannosidase | *MANBA,* 4q24 |
| α-Fucosides, glycolipids | α-Fucosidosis | α-Fucosidase | *FUCA1,* 1p36.1 |
| α-*N*-Acetylgalactosaminide | Schindler–Kanzaki disease | α-*N*-Acetylgalactosaminidase | *NAGA,* 22q13.2 |
| Sialyloligosaccharides | Sialidosis (Mucolipidosis I) | α-Neuraminidase | *NEU1,* 6p21.33 |
| Aspartylglucosamine | Aspartylglucosaminuria | Aspartylglucosaminidase | *AGA,* 4q34–35 |

**Table 1. (Continued)**

| Stored Substrate | Disease | Enzyme/Protein Deficiency | Gene Locus |
|---|---|---|---|
| MULTIPLE ENZYME DEFICIENCIES | | | |
| Glycolipids, oligosaccharides | Mucolipidosis II (I-cell disease); mucolipidosis III (pseudo-Hurler polydystrophy) three – complementation groups | *N*-Acetylglucosamine-1-phosphotransferase | Mucolipidoses II, IIIA/B: α/β subunit (*GNPTAB*) on 12q23.2; Mucolipidosis IIIC: γ subunit (*GNPTG*) mutations on 16p13.3 |
| Glycolipids, gangliosides, phospholipids | Mucolipidosis IV | Mucolipin-1 | (*MCOLN1*), 19p13.2 |
| | Galactosialidosis | Protective protein/cathepsin A | *CTSA,* 20q13.12 |
| Sulfatides, glycolipids, glycosaminoglycans | Multiple sulfatases | Sulfatase-modifying factor 1(SUMF-1) | *SUMF1,* 3p26.1 |
| LIPIDS | | | |
| Cholesterol esters | Wolman disease, cholesteryl ester storage disease | Lysosomal acid lipase | *LIPA,* 10q23.2–q23.3 |
| Cholesterol, sphingomyelin | Niemann–Pick disease type C | NPC1; NPC2 | (*NPC1*), 18q11.2; (*NPC2*), 14q24.3 |
| MONOSACCHARIDES/AMINO ACID MONOMERS | | | |
| Sialic acid, glucuronic acid | Salla disease, infantile free sialic acid storage disease | Sialin | (*SLC17A5*), 6q13 |
| Cystine | Cystinosis | Cystinosin | ***(CTNS*),** 17p13.2 |
| PEPTIDES | | | |
| Bone proteins | Pyknodysostosis | Cathepsin K | (*CTSK*), 1q21 |
| S-ACYLATED PROTEINS | | | |
| Palmitoylated proteins | Infantile neuronal ceroid lipofuscinosis | Palmitoyl-protein thioesterase 1 | (*PPT1*), 1p32 |
| Pepstatin-insensitive lysosomal peptidase | Late infantile neuronal ceroid lipofuscinosis | Tripeptidyl peptidase | (*TPP1*), 11p15 |

Incidentally, in the first section which deals with customary roles of the lysosome, diseases or gene mutations that have an impact on these processes are mentioned briefly. In some cases, examples given may not be a lysosomal storage disease; these were chosen as they provide insights relating to the consequences of certain mutations on pathways that entangle the lysosome.

There are at least 50 different lysosomal storage disorders. In the pre-molecular era, conditions were grouped according to the biochemical composition of the stored substrate (e.g., sphingolipidosis, glycosamino-glycans, etc.) (Table 1). More recently, diseases have been clustered based on the nature of the underlying molecular defect (i.e., mutation in the encoding enzyme, co-factor, transmembrane transport protein, etc.) (Table 2).

**Table 2. Lysosomal storage disorders, listed according to underlying cause**

| Etiology | Disease (Examples) |
|---|---|
| Single hydrolytic enzyme deficiency | Gaucher disease<br>Tay–Sachs disease<br>Niemann–Pick A/B disease |
| Single protease enzyme deficiency | Late infantile neuronal ceroid lipofuscinosis (tripeptidyl peptidase) |
| Co-factor/activator protein deficiency | Gaucher disease variant (saposin C)<br>Tay–Sachs disease variant ($GM_2$ activator) |
| Multiple enzyme deficiencies | Galactosialidosis (PPCA) (protective protein/cathepsin A)<br>Multiple sulfatase deficiency (SUMF-1)<br>I-cell disease (mucolipidosis II) |
| Membrane protein defect | Juvenile neuronal ceroid lipofuscinosis (battenin) |
| Small-molecule transport protein | Cystinosis (cystinosin)<br>Sialic acid storage disorders (sialin) |
| Endocytosis, membrane–vesicle trafficking defect | Mucolipidosis IV (mucolipin)<br>Danon disease (LAMP-2)<br>Niemann–Pick disease type C (NPC1/NPC2) |

It has been said that every book is in some sense a collective undertaking, upheld by the intellectual endeavours and accumulated wisdom of past and present generations. In closing, I would like to pay tribute to those individuals who have shaped my thinking about lysosomal storage disorders; these include not only colleagues, but most especially patients from whom I have gained practical experience in both the science and art of medicine. In the first instance, there are too many and I would not like to offend any by their inadvertent exclusion. In the latter case, I am obliged to maintain patient privacy and confidentially. Altogether, let those concerned be assured of my profound gratitude.

*Chapter 1*

# Introduction and General Aspects

A central role in homeostasis has been ascribed to the lysosome, which previously had been viewed mainly as the terminal compartment ('wastebin') of metabolism where cellular debris was directed for disposal. This historical perspective reflected a time, when characterization of disease was largely driven by anatomical findings, and subsequently identififcation of the underlying enzyme defects and associated substrate deposits.

More recently, the application of molecular genetic techniques has led to increased understanding of putative downstream mechanisms of disease. Moreover, there is recognition of the novel role the lysosome plays in nutrient sensing and its interactions with various systems involved with maintaining cellular homeostasis, such as the ubiquitin-proteasome pathway and autophagy.

Recent studies have focused attention on a network responsible for the coordinated expression of proteins targeted to the lysosome and engaged in lysosomal biogenesis. As it turns out, the relevant factors are involved with transcription not only of lysosomal-related genes but those involved with the process of autophagy and exocytosis as well [1]. These homeostatic activities, including the innate inflammatory response and cell death pathways, have been shown to be perturbed in several LSDs; however, their precise mechanistic links with the accumulating substrate remain to be more fully elucidated. Most studies have been undertaken in animal models and in fibroblasts obtained from affected patients; in the latter case, it is uncertain whether any of the observed findings are generalizable to all affected tissue types, such as brain tissue (i.e., neurons, astrocytes).

Thus, the lysosome and related organelles may be conceived as components of a dynamic system of compartments, integrating trafficking routes and sorting and recycling/clearance machineries (*schematically represented in* Figure 1.1).

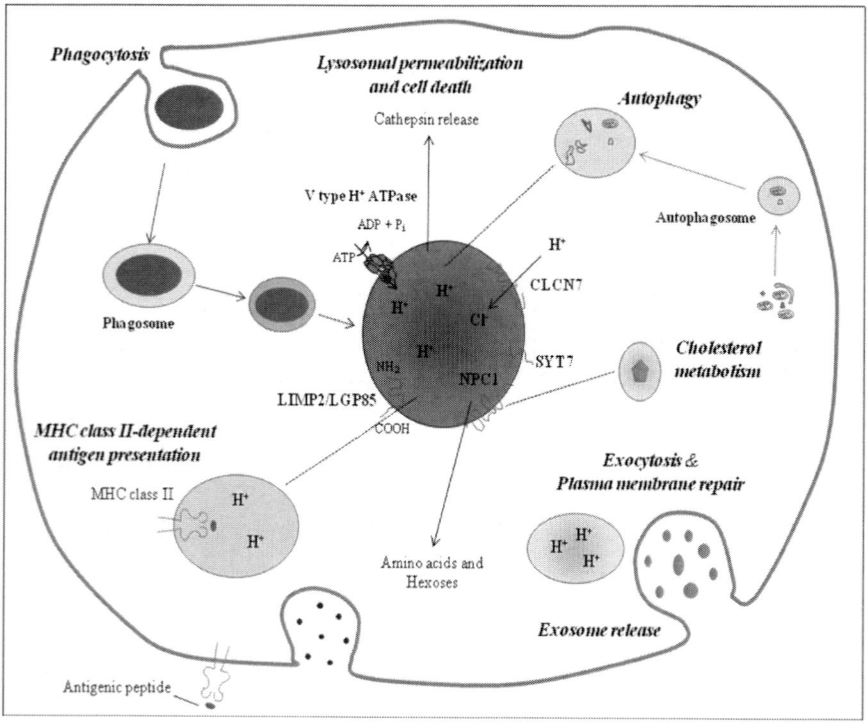


Figure 1.1. The lysosome, its central role and involvement in several cellular processes.

## 1.1. Lysosome: General Attributes

First described by Christian de Duve in 1955, lysosomes are small, spherical intracellular bodies with amorphous, electron-dense cores and a single limiting membrane enclosing an acidic (pH 4.8-5.0) milieu.

Lysosomes are filled with an array of hydrolases that can degrade all cellular macromolecules, which are directed to the lysosome for degradation by phagocytosis, endocytosis and autophagy (Figure 1.2; supplementary information noted in Box 1.1).

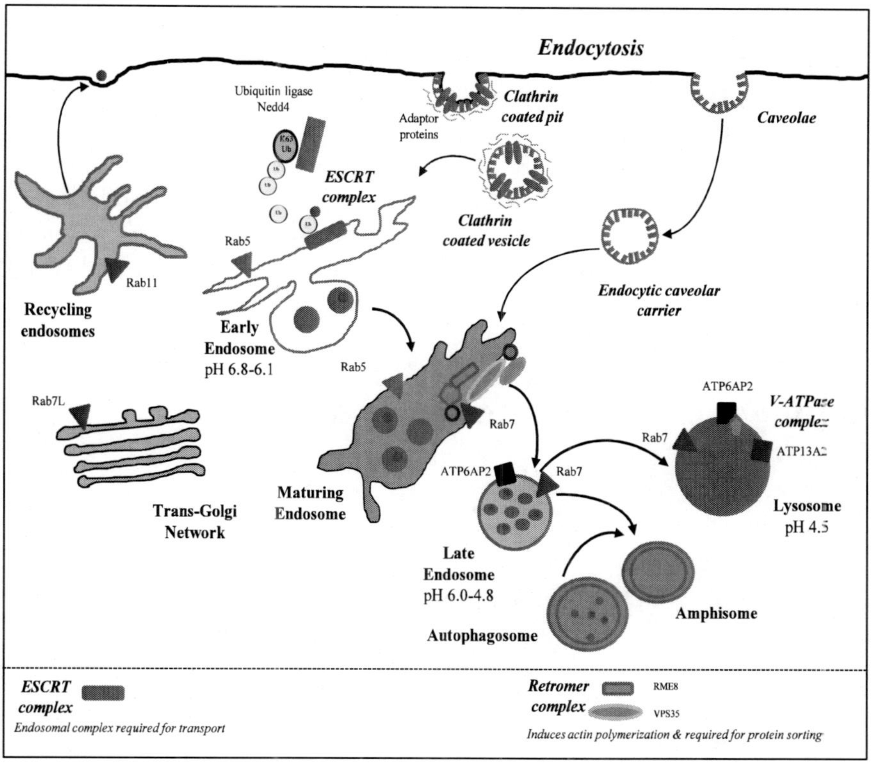


Figure 1.2. The endosome-lysosomal system and autophagy[1].

---

[1] The Endosomal Sorting Complexes required for Transport (ESCRT) plays a key role in the formation of late endosomes/multi-vesicular bodies, through its ability to induce a topologically unique membrane bending and scission reaction away from the cytoplasm. The ESCRT machinery include five distinct complexes (ESCRT-0, -I, -II, -III and the Vps4 complex); which have tasks (from interaction with ubiquitinated membrane proteins to membrane deformation and abscission), allowing flexibility in the integration of three different biological processes, with which its has been implicated: multivesicular body formation, cytokinesis and HIV budding.

The retromer complex is a component of the intracellular trafficking mechanism sorting cargo from the endosomes to the trans-Golgi network or to the cell surface. Components of the retromer complex and members of the vacuolar protein sorting 10 (Vps10) family of receptors play pleiotropic functions in protein trafficking and intracellular/intercellular signalling in neuronal and non-neuronal cells and are primary

Lysosomes also take part in transactions with other 'independent' compartments, such as the endoplasmic reticulum and mitochondria. Among other cellular functions, these inter-organelle exchanges involve the transfer and metabolism of lipids and the modulation of calcium fluxes. A disruption of this fusion or transient communication between organelles may underlie defects of autophagy, as seen with certain lysosomal disorders such as Niemann-Pick disease type C[2].

In addition to animal models of disease (*see* Box 1.2), the generation of induced pluripotent stem cells (iPSCs) from affected patients' fibroblasts and subsequent differentiation of these stem cells to specific types of interest has become a powerful tool for human disease modelling and therapeutic screening.

## a. Biogenesis and Interactions with Other Organelles

Although initially viewed as a terminus of metabolism, fed by endocytosis and used mainly for macromolecule degradation, lysosomes are now recognized as dynamic organelles with multiple roles [2, 3]. Moreover, lysosome-related organelles (such as melanosomes) exist in specialized cells to serve specific functions (e.g., production of the pigment melanin) [4]; typically co-existing with conventional lysosomes.

Endosomes form to deliver ingested molecules from the extracellular space for degradation; acquiring lysosomal proteins and an acidic pH in the course of their maturation from early to late endosomes. These transformative processes are accompanied by vesicle trafficking, protein sorting and targeted degradation of sorted cargo. These processes are regulated by the Rab family of small GTPases; and different Rab proteins serve as markers of distinct endosomal compartments.

---

cargos of the retromer complex, which have been implicated as genetic risk factors for sporadic and autosomal dominant forms of several neurodegenerative diseases, including Alzheimer disease, frontotemporal lobar degeneration, and Parkinson disease. Additionally, members of the Vps10 receptor family (sortilin, SorL1, SorCS1, SorCS2, and SorCS3) modulate neurotrophic signalling pathways.

[2] Niemann-Pick disease type C is a neurodegenerative disorder. Mutations of NPC1 account for ~95% of cases. NPC1 and NPC2 are proteins located in late endosomes/lysosomes; these proteins are thought to work in tandem and mediate the egress of cholesterol and other lipid cargo from lysosomes.

Cytosolic proteins requiring intralysosomal cleavage are provided to endosomes by the *Endosomal Sorting Complexes required for Transport* (ESCRT) pathway [5]. ESCRT complexes package ubiquitinated proteins into vesicles, formed by the inward budding of the endosomal limiting membrane. Dysregulation of ESCRT-mediated proteostasis in glial cells have been implicated in Alzheimer disease [6]. Endocytosed calcium and calmodulin are believed to play a critical role in these events, and also with the reformation of lysosomes and the dynamic equilibrium of organelles in the late endocytic pathway. Small molecular products of lysosomal digestion are released into the cytosol via transport proteins (e.g., sialin, cystinosin) (Figure 1.3). Exit of digested material from the lysosome also implicate exocytosis in some cases.

In parallel, the formation of multivesicular (MV) bodies and intraluminal vesicles can occur, independent of ESCRT involvement. This process engages two enzymes in the limiting membranes of MV bodies, i.e., neutral sphingomyelinase and phospholipase A2; which facilitate the generation of lipids to induce inward budding [3].

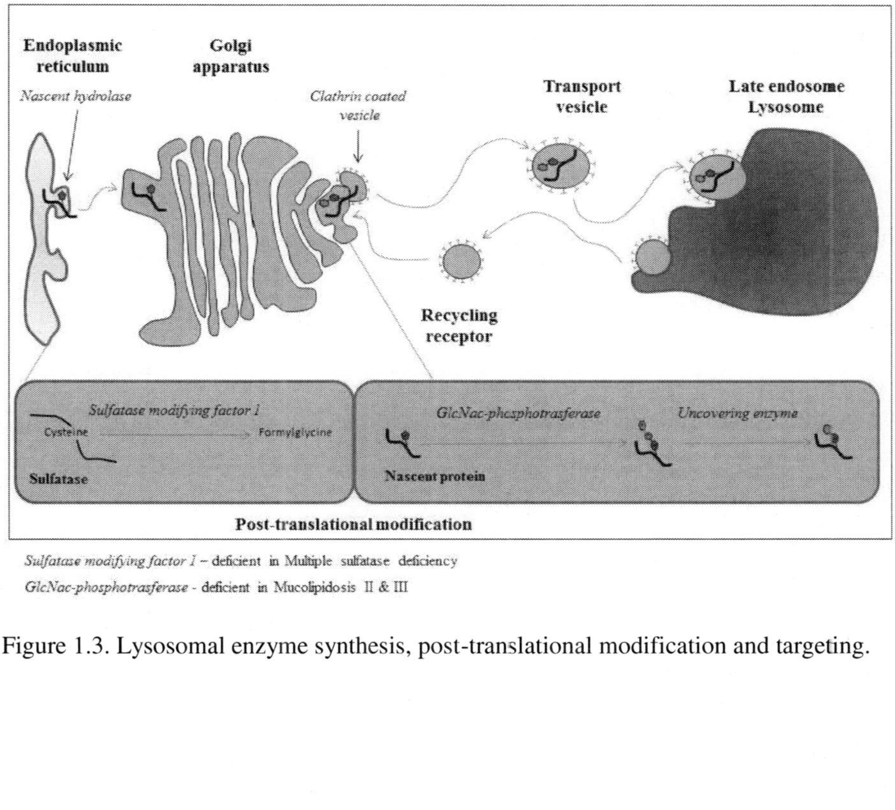


Figure 1.3. Lysosomal enzyme synthesis, post-translational modification and targeting.

A glycoconjugate coat is present on the inside of the lysosomal membrane ("lysosomal glycocalyx"), with the lysosomal associated membrane proteins LAMP-1 and LAMP-2 as major constituents [7]. It is this inner lining of the lysosomal membrane, with a thickness ranging from 5 to 12 nm, which prevents autodigestion; essentially helping to contain an acidified environment replete with hydrolases and other effector molecules, such as cathepins. Glycoprotein membrane coats also can be observed in endosomes, autophagosomes and secretory granules; likely helping to prevent leakage of organelle contents into the cytoplasm. Increased lysosomal membrane permeabilization and the release of effector molecules are engaged in cell death (*discussed in Chapter 2*).

The LAMP family is characterized by a conserved domain of 150 to 200 amino acids, which forms a novel β-prism fold, made up of two β-sheets bent by β-bulges and connected by a disulfide bond. The flexible loops and a hydrophobic pocket are thought to represent possible sites of molecular interaction. LAMP proteins are important regulators of lysosome fusion with phagosomes and autophagosomes, and LAMP-2 has been implicated in cholesterol transport from the lysosome. Deficiency of LAMP-2 (lgp110, CD107b) causes Danon disease [8], a neuromuscular glycogen storage disorder characterized by a defect of chaperone-mediated autophagy.

### *a.1. Autophagy*

Autophagy, a lysosomal-mediated cellular degradation pathway for the selective removal of damaged cytosolic proteins and organelles (e.g., damaged mitochondria), encompass three main pathways: (1) chaperone-mediated autophagy (CMA); (2) microautophagy (resulting from direct invagination of lysosomal membranes to engulf cellular components); and (3) macroautophagy [9]. Macroautophagy, the most well-studied, consist of two consecutive stages, involving the formation of the double membrane autophagosome and its subsequent fusion with the lysosome (*see* Figure 1.4). Autophagosomes are transferred along microtubules in a dynein-dependent manner to bring them into close contact with lysosomes.

In CMA, cytosolic substrate proteins (e.g., α-synuclein aggregates) are tagged (via a recognition sequence: KFERQ or KFERQ-like motif) by heat shock cognate protein 70 (hsc70) complex and subsequently bound to monomers of LAMP-2A; which then multimerizes to form a unit required for α-synuclein transmembrane import into the lysosome [9]. Membrane-associated molecules of hsc70 actively disassemble LAMP-2A into monomers to initiate a new cycle of binding and translocation. α-synuclein mutants lacking the CMA motif or siRNA-mediated knockdown of LAMP2 lead to slower turnover of wild-type α-synuclein.

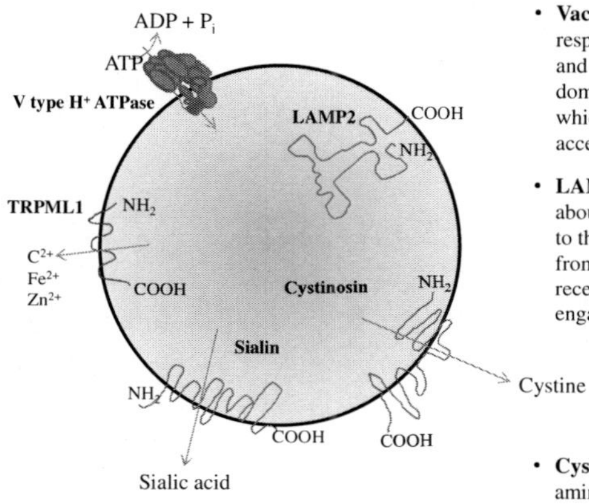


- **Vacuolar type $H^+$ ATPase**: multisubunit complex responsible for acidification of endosomes, lysosomes, and other intracellular organelles. Cytosolic catalytic domain consists of 3 A subunits and 3 B subunits, which bind and hydrolyze ATP, as well as regulatory accessory subunits including C, D and E.
- **LAMP2**: glycoprotein consisting of polypeptides of about 40 kD, with 16 to 20 N-linked saccharides attached to the core polypeptides; protects lysosomal membrane from proteolytic enzymes within lysosomes; acts as a receptor for proteins imported into lysosomes; also engaged in vesicle fusion and cholesterol homeostasis
- **Cystinosin**: putative cystine transporter (comprised 367 amino acids, 7 transmembrane domains)
- **Sialin (SLC17A5)**: in lysosomes, acts as an $H^+$-coupled sialic acid exporter. In CNS synaptic vesicles, responsible for vesicular storage and subsequent exocytosis of aspartate and glutamate
- **TRPML1**: principal $C^{2+}$ release channel in lysosomes

Figure 1.4. Lysosomal membrane proteins/transporters.

Autophagy is tightly associated with cellular survival, and its activation/ inhibition is influenced by cellular stress/starvation. The mammalian target of rapamycin complex 1 (mTORC1) exerts an inhibitory effect on autophagy, mediated via phosphorylation of the autophagy regulator ULK1 (*see* Box 1.3). Deficiency of progranulin has been shown to lead to decreased mTORC1 activity, associated with an increase of lysosomal biogenesis and the expression of autophagosome-related genes [10]. Homozygous mutations in the progranulin gene (*PGRN*) have been found in two siblings suffering from a newly described type of adult onset neuronal ceroid lipofuscinosis.

Interestingly, the production of progranulin is increased in activated microglia after traumatic brain injury.

### a.1.1. Aggrephagy

Aggrephagy is a cargo-specific subtype of autophagy important for degrading ubiquitinated target proteins through the lysosome. Defects of aggrephagy have been implicated in amyotrophic lateral sclerosis and frontotemporal dementia; diseases characterized by altered protein clearance and tissue deposits [11]. TAR DNA binding protein and fused in sarcoma (FUS), which are implicated in these disorders, are RNA processing proteins whose dysfunction impacts on global cellular RNA regulation. TAR DNA binding protein and FUS both bind and regulate key aggrephagy-related genes; dysfunction of aggrephagy leads to cytoplasmic relocalization and aggregation of TAR DNA binding protein.

### *a.2. Targeting of Nascent Proteins to the Lysosomal Compartment*

Transmembrane proteins (i.e., localized to the lysosomal membrane, such as LIMP1) have sorting signals in their cytosolic domains. On the other hand, nascent soluble enzymes (e.g., α-galactosidase A, galactocerebrosidase) that ultimately reside within the lysosome are tagged with mannose-6-phosphate (M6P) [12] (Figure 1.4 and Box 1.4). Marked proteins are sorted in the Golgi compartment by M6P receptors, and exit the trans-Golgi network as clathrin-coated vesicles which fuse with endosomes. In I-cell disease (mucolipidosis-II[3]), defective post-translational modification of several lysosomal hydrolases and absence of the appropriate M6P tag lead to their extra-cellular release and consequent intralysosomal accumulation of their corresponding substrates [13].

There are other routes (besides uptake via cation-independent M6P receptors) which enable newly synthesized proteins to gain access to the lysosome [14]. For instance, the nonenzymatic sphingolipid activator protein (prosaposin) traffics to lysosomes through the sorting receptor sortilin (neurotensin receptor-3); whilst the enzyme β–glucosidase (encoded by *GBA*) transits via the lysosomal integral membrane protein-2 (LIMP-2) interaction.[4,5]

---

[3] Mucolipidosis-II (and its attenuated form, ML-III) is caused by a deficiency of UDP-GlcNAc:lysosomal enzyme GlcNAc-1-phosphotransferase, which is responsible for tagging lysosomal enzymes with M6P. In an affected ML-II animal model, extracellular cathepsin K activity has been shown to promote abnormal bone and cartilage development by disrupting the balance of TGFß-related signalling during chondrogenesis. This defect may underlie features of dysostosis seen in this condition.

[4] Wild type *LIMP-2* undergoes proteolytic cleavage by lysosomal cysteine proteases, mainly cathepsin-F. Mutations in the gene encoding cathepsin-F (CTSF) have been associated with type-B-Kufs-disease, an adult form of neuronal ceroid lipofuscinosis. Remarkably, *LIMP-2* (SCARB2) has also been identified as a receptor for enterovirus 71 uptake.

Sortilin, a member of the receptor family of vacuolar protein sorting-10 (VPS10), has been implicated as a genetic risk factor for neurodegenerative diseases such as Alzheimer disease, frontotemporal lobar degeneration, and Parkinson disease [15].

LIMP-2 has been shown to be essential not only for (β-glucosidase (glucocerebrosidase) lysosomal targeting; it is also engaged in α-synuclein clearance (through CMA). These observations are of interest, given the association between *GBA* mutations and the risk for developing Parkinson disease.

## b. Lysosomal Acidification

Acidification of the intralysosomal microenvironment is achieved through the action of rotary motors (vacuolar ATPases, V-ATPases); made up of two sectors: a V1 catalytic domain and VO membrane domain. Intracellular V-ATPases ($H^+$-ATPases) are versatile, with broader functions and involvement in several cellular processes such as receptor-mediated endocytosis (occurring on the plasma membrane), intracellular membrane trafficking, prohormone processing, protein degradation (within the lysosome) and neurotransmitter uptake (in secretory granules). V-ATPases have also been shown to be required for sensing amino acids inside the lysosomal lumen, which is a factor in mTORC1 activation (*see* Box 1.3).

In general, V-ATPases use the energy derived from ATP hydrolysis to shuttle various substrates, ranging from cations and heavy metals to lipids, across biological membranes and against their concentration gradients [16]. Chloride channel interacting protein (ClC) and $Na^+/K^+$ channels/transporters contribute to acidification by providing counter ions. V-ATPase differs from other ATPase (such as plasma membrane $Na^+/K^+$-ATPase and sarcoplasmic reticulum $Ca^{2+}$-ATPase), in that it does not require a coupled influx of permanent anions.

Acidification of the endosome by V-ATPase allows for release of the endocytosed ligand, which enables recycling of the corresponding receptor back to the membrane. This process is regulated by Rab4 and Rab11. Budding of endosomal carrier vesicles and multivesicular bodies are also dependent on

[5] Mutations of LIMP-2 have been associated with a separate disorder: autosomal recessive myoclonic epilepsy and glomerulosclerosis.

an acidic environment. Vesicle fusion with pre-existing early endosomes occurs under the direction of Rab5. The maturation from early to late endosomes is accompanied by the transition from association with Rab5 to Rab7.

In the lysosome, acidification activates cathepsins and other degradative enzymes. Interestingly, enveloped viruses and bacterial toxins (e.g., diphtheria toxin) have been shown to enter cells via endocytosis; the low pH generated by the V-ATPase within the endosomes causes the viral coat to fuse with the endosomal membrane, releasing viral mRNAs into the cytoplasm, propagating the infectious process. Similarly, the acidic environment induces the diphtheria toxin B chain to form a pore in the membrane that facilitates the entry of the A chain into the cytoplasm.

Loss of the $H^+$-ATPase a3 subunit or ClC-1 (or its beta-subunit Ostm1), impairs lysosomal acidification [17]. The associated defect in proteolysis, which is seen in these conditions, causes a defect in bone resorption (osteopetrosis). Recently, defects of presenilin- 1 (PS-1, mutations of which lead to familial Alzheimer disease) has been shown to lead to a disruption of lysosomal acidification and proteolysis, associated with inhibition of autophagy. These changes have been attributed to impaired glycosylation and instability of the V-ATPase V0a1 subunit, causing deficient lysosomal V-ATPase assembly and function [18]. The elevated lysosomal pH in the PS-1 knockout cells was found to induce abnormal $Ca^{2+}$ efflux from lysosomes mediated by TRPML1[6], resulting in elevated cytosolic $Ca^{2+}$. Remarkably, normalizing lysosomal pH in affected cells using acidic nanoparticles restored normal lysosomal proteolysis, autophagy, and $Ca^{2+}$ homeostasis; but correcting lysosomal $Ca^{2+}$ deficits alone neither re-acidified lysosomes nor reversed proteolytic and autophagic deficits.

Of note: V-ATPase assembly integral membrane protein VMA21 is an essential chaperone for V-ATPase. Mutations of the encoding gene have been identified as the cause of X-linked myopathy with excessive autophagy [19].

[6] TRPML1 (mucolipin-1) is a cation channel protein; mutations of its encoding gene is the cause of Mucolipidosis type IV (ML-IV), a neurodegenerative lysosomal storage disorder characterized by impaired motor and cognitive development, progressive loss of vision and gastric achlorhydria. White matter abnormalities and a hypoplastic corpus callosum are the major hallmarks of ML-IV brain pathology. Defects of brain myelination have been attributed to deficient maturation and loss of oligodendrocytes.

## c. Coordinated Gene Expression and the Secretory-Endosomal-Autophagy-Lysosomal-Exocytic (SEALE) Network

The degradation of macromolecules within the lysosomes entails sequential substrate cleavage down to its fundamental units; a process which necessitates the coordinated expression of the relevant hydrolases. Indeed, concentration of these hydrolases within the lysosomes, which show little to no sequence homology, suggest convergent evolution.

Co-expression analysis of lysosomal genes (using publicly available microarray data) led to recognition that the promoter of genes encoding lysosomal hydrolases contained an E-box (i.e., a palindromic 10-base site that is a target for the b-HLH transcription factor). This observation indicated these genes were highly co-expressed; subsequent studies closed the loop on this issue by showing that regulation of lysosomal gene expression was mediated by a master transcription factor EB (TFEB), which belongs to the MiT subfamily of b-HLH transcription factor EB and is a constituent of the CLEAR[7] network [20]. Ensuing studies revealed TFEB is also involved with regulation of autophagy-related genes.

A combination of genomic approaches, including: (1) ChIP-seq (chromatin immunoprecipitate sequencing) analysis, (2) the profiling of TFEB-mediated transcriptional induction, (3) genome-wide mapping of TFEB target sites, and (4) recursive expression meta-analysis of TFEB targets, has enabled the identification of 471 TFEB direct targets [21]. A systematic approach to ascertain relevant cellular pathways involved remains to be done.

TFEB is regulated by phosphorylation, which is mediated by mTORC1 at the lysosomal surface (*see* Box 1.3 and Figure 1.5). Conditions resulting in inhibition of mTOR, such as starvation and lysosomal stress, or administration of catalytic inhibitors of mTOR (e.g., PP242 and Torin 1) promote TFEB dephosphorylation and its subsequent nuclear translocation. This leads to transcription of several genes encoding lysosomal hydrolases and those implicated in autophagy. These factors constitute the CLEAR network; used

---

[7] CLEAR (which stands for Coordinated Lysosomal Expression and Regulation) represents a comprehensive system which is involved with regulation of the expression, import and activity of lysosomal enzymes that control the degradation of various substrates such as proteins, glycosaminoglycans, sphingolipids and glycogen. This network has also been found to be engaged in the regulation of additional processes, including autophagy, exo- and endo-cytosis, phagocytosis and the immune response.

by the cell to recycle components required to feed the synthetic pathway (*discussed further in the succeeding section*).

Recent studies have shown another transcription factor E3 (TFE3, a member of the same MiTF/TFE family) also regulates lysosomal homeostasis; involved with inducing the expression of genes encoding proteins involved in autophagy and lysosomal biogenesis (as shown in ARPE-19 cells in response to starvation and lysosomal stress) [21]. As with TFEB, mTORC1-mediated phosphorylation of TFE3 results in its retention in the cytosol through its interaction with the cytosolic chaperone 14-3-3. After starvation, TFE3 is rapidly dephosphorylated, activated and subsequently translocated to the nucleus; where it binds to CLEAR (Coordinated Lysosomal Expression and Regulation) elements (i.e., E-box) present in the promoter region of many lysosomal- and autophagy-related genes, thereby inducing lysosomal and autophagosome biogenesis.

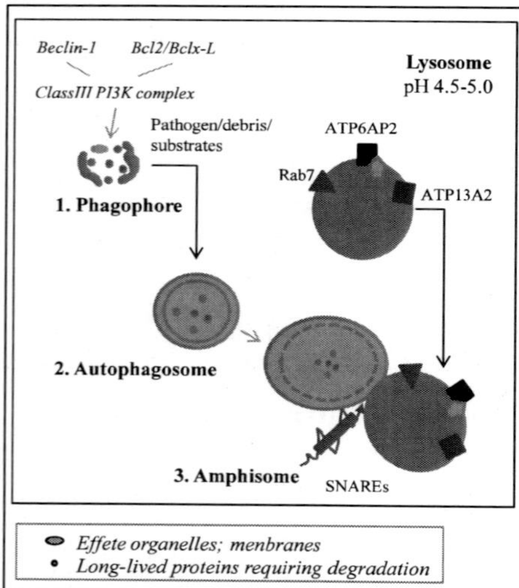


| | |
|---|---|
| VPS34 | vacuolar protein sorting-34 |
| PI-3-P | phosphatidylinositol-3-phosphate |
| PE | phosphatidylethanolamine |
| LC3 | micro-tubule associated protein-light chain 3 |

- Early phase
  - Induction stimulated by pathogen/substrate recognition receptor (PRR) ligand *(capture and degradation of pathogens/substrate)*
  - Vesicle nucleation, assembly of phagophores, facilitated by a protein complex consisting of VPS34 and Beclin-1 *(which initiates phosphorylation of PI-1-P)*
  - Autophagophore elongation, via ubiquitin E3-ligase complex (Atg7, Atg12 and Atg16L1) *(conjugates PE to micro-tubule associated protein-light chain 3);* p62 binds to LC3-PE, fixing it in the inner and outer membranes of autophagosome
- Late phase
  - Fusion with lysosome (autophagolysosome formation), involving Stx17 as the first SNARE (soluble N-ethylmaleide-sensitive factor attachment protein receptor)

Figure 1.5. Stages of Macro-autophagy and Autophagosome-Lysosome fusion.

## d. Lysosomal Nutrient Sensing (LyNus) and mTORC Regulation

The involvement of lysosomes with the degradation of macromolecules generated from cellular turnover has, in many peoples' minds, led to a limited view of lysosomes as an organelle mainly responsible for the clearance or elimination of various substrates. More recently, it has been recognized that lysosomes also may have a critical role in the recycling of cellular materials, linked to autophagy and the balance between 'fed' or 'fasted' state (i.e., a nutrient sensing role); processes partly regulated by mTORC1 (*see* Box 1.3, Figure 1.5). This phenomenon may be a means of conserving energy, as it minimizes the need to synthesize essential precursors.

The mechanistic target of rapamycin complex 1 (mTORC1) is known to integrate the presence of growth factors, energy levels, glucose and amino acids. Studies have shown mTORC1 is activated at the surface of lysosomes, linked with a complex (LyNUS machinery, *see* Figure 1.5) involved with the monitoring of amino acid availability within the lysosomal lumen [22]. Phosphorylation at Thr-2446, Ser-2448 and Ser-2481 within the kinase catalytic (KIN) domain of mTORC, are correlated with overall higher levels of its activity. Activation of mTORC leads to phosphorylation of ribosomal protein S6 kinase (S6K), eukaryotic initiation factor 4E-binding protein 1 (4E-BP1), ULK1, and the transcription factor TFEB; which leads to enhanced translation and cell growth (mediated by S6K and 4E-BP1), suppression of autophagy (ULK1), and retention of TFEB in the cytoplasm as an inactive form (bound to 14-3-3 chaperone protein).

Regulation of mTORC1 can be mediated by: 1) growth factors which stimulate AKT, which - in turn - phosphorylates (thereby inhibiting) the tuberous sclerosis complex (TSC); (2) activation of AMP-Kinase in response to a low energy status; and (3) activation of suppressor genes (such as PTEN, AMPK, LKB1)[8]. These various pathways are involved with the inhibition of mTORC1; as noted in the preceding section, this leads to the nuclear translocation of TFEB (and TFE3), which promotes the transcription of autophagy- and lysosomal-related genes (*see* Figure 1.6).

[8] Conversely, oncogenes (such as class I *PI3K*, *Ras*, *Rheb*, and *AKT*) activate mTOR and inhibit autophagy. PI3Ks mostly generate phospholipids serving to transduce signals generated by receptor tyrosine kinases and G protein-coupled receptors.

It has been hypothesized that mTORC1 may be differentially regulated by specific amino acids. Indeed, it has been demonstrated the amino acids leucine and glutamine stimulates mTORC1 by Rag GTPase-dependent and -independent mechanisms, respectively [22]. Adenosine diphosphate ribosylation factor-1 GTPase has also been identified as necessary for this process to occur.

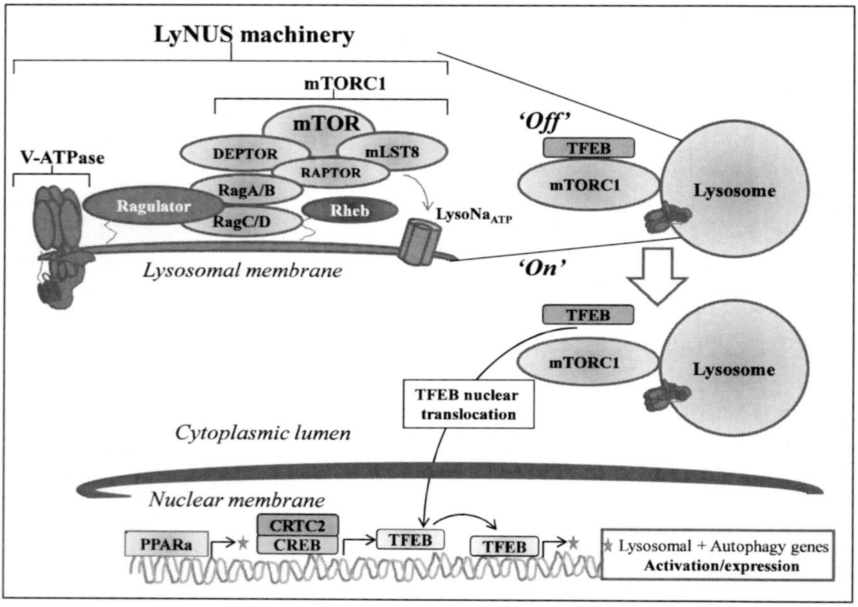


**RAPTOR:** regulatory-associated protein of mTOR **DEPTOR**: DEP domain-containing mTOR

Figure 1.6. LyNus, mTORC1 and TFEB.

Studies have found glutamine promoted mTORC1 translocation to the lysosomal surface in RagA- and RagB-knockout cells, in a reaction which required V-ATPase (involved with 'inside-outside' amino acid signalling). Notably, *in vitro* studies have shown loss of RagA and RagB (RagA/B) in cardiomyocytes results in hypertrophic cardiomyopathy which mimics a lysosomal storage disease.

Recently, the human member 9 of the solute carrier family 38 (SLC38A9) has been identified as a lysosomal membrane-resident protein engaged in amino acid transport [23]. Functional proteomic analysis has established SLC38A9 is an integral part of the Ragulator-Rag GTPases machinery, involved with mTORC1 regulation. Gain of SLC38A9 function rendered cells resistant to amino acid withdrawal, whereas loss of SLC38A9 expression impaired amino acid-induced mTORC1 activation.

## e. Intracellular Calcium Signalling

Changes in the intracellular concentration of calcium ($Ca^{2+}$) are well-orchestrated, as $Ca^{2+}$ is an integral cationic messenger and a component of the signal transduction pathway; in a process which involves "acidic $Ca^{2+}$ stores", such as acidocalcisomes, the endo-lysosomal system, lysosome-related organelles, secretory vesicles and the Golgi complex [24].

Incidentally, $Ca^{2+}$ uptake into acidic $Ca^{2+}$ stores is driven by $Ca^{2+}$-ATPases and $Ca^{2+}/H^+$ exchangers. In animal cells, the $Ca^{2+}$-mobilizing messenger nicotinamide adenine dinucleotide phosphate (NAADP) plays a central role in mediating $Ca^{2+}$ signals from acidic $Ca^{2+}$ stores through activation of two-pore channels (TCPs) [25]. These signals are important for several physiological processes including muscle contraction and differentiation. Inositol trisphosphate and ryanodine receptors, which are traditionally viewed as endoplasmic reticulum $Ca^{2+}$ release channels, are also involved with mobilizing $Ca^{2+}$ from acidic stores.

Neurons possess an elaborate system of endo-lysosomes with readily releasable stores of intracellular $Ca^{2+}$. Recent studies in primary cultured neurons have shown $Ca^{2+}$ released from acidic stores triggered calcium influx across the plasma membrane (a phenomenon termed "acidic store-operated calcium entry", aSOCE) [26]. [aSOCE is functionally distinct from store-operated calcium release and entry involving the endoplasmic reticulum.]

aSOCE is regulated at least in part by exocytotic insertion of N-type $Ca^{2+}$ channels into plasma membranes through LAMP1-dependent lysosome exocytosis. siRNA knockdown of LAMP1 or Rab27a, both of which are key proteins involved in lysosome exocytosis, has been found to attenuate aSOCE.

Recently, lysosomal $Ca^{2+}$ release through mucolipin 1 (MCOLN1, TRPML1) has been shown to activate calcineurin, which subsequently binds and dephosphorylates TFEB; in turn promoting the nuclear translocation of TFEB and the transcription of autophagy- and lysosome-related genes [27].

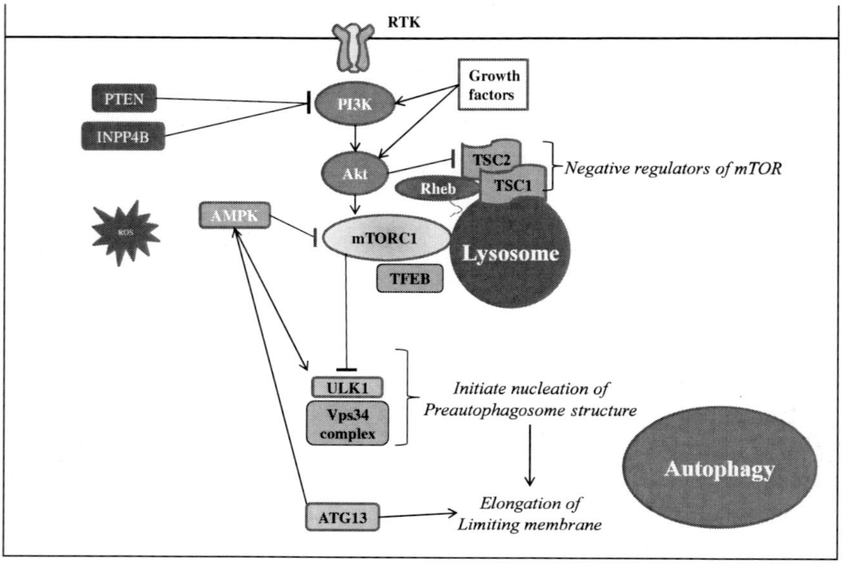


**Rheb:** Ras homolog enriched in brain; mTOR activator.

Figure 1.7. mTORC1 and regulatory factors.

## f. Plasma Membrane Repair

Lysosomes have been linked with the repair of the plasma membrane, which is essential in restoring cellular homeostasis and ensuring cell survival after injury. Calcium-dependent exocytosis of lysosomes is an important early step in the plasma membrane repair (or re-sealing) process; defects of which have been observed in cells bearing mutations responsible for lysosomal diseases such as Niemann-Pick disease type A (acid sphingomyelinase deficiency) and Chediak-Higashi syndrome.[9]

It has been suggested, other $Ca^{2+}$-dependent cytosolic proteins, such as calpain, annexins and/or transglutaminases, are be involved in generating a barrier to cytosolic loss at wound sites [28]. Models of plasma membrane repair mechanisms, which are postulated to be dependent on local increases in

[9] Chediak-Higashi syndrome is a rare, autosomal recessive congenital immunodeficiency caused by mutations in CHS1, a gene encoding a putative lysosomal trafficking protein. In the majority of patients, this disorder is typically characterized by infantile-onset hemophagocytic lymphohistiocytosis (HLH), which is lethal unless allogeneic transplantation is performed.

intracellular $Ca^{2+}$ at injury sites include the "lipid-patch", "endocytic removal", and "macro-vesicle shedding".

Normally, the lysosomal enzyme acid sphingomyelinase is released following plasma membrane injury; this leads to the generation of ceramide on the cell surface, which triggers endocytosis and removal of the injured membrane section and its subsequent repair [29]. It is possible other lysosomal hydrolases are involved with plasma membrane repair, but this remains to be confirmed. Membrane-remodeling by the ESCRT complex has also been shown to participate in small-wound repair.

Incidentally, mutations of caveolin (integral membrane proteins forming a component of discrete membrane microdomains) and cavins (another set of protein that form a scaffold to support the cytosolic face of caveolae) are associated with defects of skeletal and cardiac muscle – tissues subjected to mechanical stress and likely require plasma membrane remodelling on a regular basis [30].

## g. Antigen Presentation

Dendritic cells (DCs) are professional antigen-presenting cells tasked with activation of immune responses; initiated by the priming of naive T cells. DCs search for and engulf pathogens in tissues that are in contact with the external environment (e.g., mucosal lining of the respiratory tract). Pathogen-specific antigens on the cell surface of DCs use Major histocompatibility complex (MHC) class II molecules; once MHC class II molecules have bound a peptide, the complex is delivered to the cell surface of DCs for presentation to $CD^{4+}$ T cells.

Intracellular antigen uptake via macropinocytosis and phagocytosis, as well as its trafficking in early endocytic vesicles are carefully regulated, and involve the small GTPase Rab5 and its effectors [31]. Details regarding the regulation of antigen delivery from early endosomes to lysosomal compartments (where the proper pH and proteases, MHC II, invariant chain, and HLA-DM proteins reside) remain to be fully elucidated.

A recent report has observed a crucial role of the small GTPase ADP-ribosylation factor-like 8b (Arl8b) in MHC II presentation in dendritic cells. Arl8b has been found to localize to MHC II compartments in DCs, involved with regulating the formation of MHC II-peptide complexes [32]. Arl8b-silenced DCs display a defect in MHC II-Ag complex formation and its delivery to the cell surface during infection, resulting in a defect in T cell recognition.

## h. DNA Processing Following Apoptosis

Apoptosis is associated with genomic DNA fragmentation into oligonucleosomes; clearance of which involves deoxyribonuclease II (DNase II, also called DNase IIα). DNase II protein is present in the lysosomes of both splenic macrophages and mononuclear cells in the bone marrow. Purification studies have revealed DNase II is found in the lysosomal fraction, which also showed the presence of lysosomal cathepsin D and acid phosphatase.

Mice deficient in DNase II die during later developmental stages; an event attributed to constitutive interferon (IFN) β production [33]. Macrophages in affected mice embryos phagocytose, but cannot digest, nuclei that are expelled from erythroid precursor cells. Further investigations have revealed mitochondrial DNA can escape from autophagic vacuoles of cardiomyocytes of affected mice, triggering a cell-autonomous activation of Toll-like receptor (TLR)-9 mediated inflammatory responses in the heart [34].

In summary, the outcome of investigations undertaken in the last decade has led to recognition of the vital role played by the lysosome in maintaining cellular homeostasis; beyond serving as a compartment for the degradation of various substrates within an acidified milieu replete with various enzymes. The next chapter focuses attention on the consequences of lysosomal dysfunction, brought on by deficiencies in acid hydrolases, their cofactors and transport proteins, which result in progressive intralysosomal substrate accumulation.

**Box 1.1. Cellular processes involving the lysosome**

*(see Figures 1.1 and 1.2)*

Lysosomes are an integral component of a network which adjusts to changing internal and external conditions to maintain cells in a dynamic equilibrium.

- **Phagocytosis**: cellular uptake pathway for particles (>0.5 μm diameter). Goal: destruction of engulfed bacteria or fungi, and signaling to mount an immune defence. Also, involved with clearance of apoptotic cells and surrounding debris. Different phagocytic pathways are stimulated by particle ligation of distinct surface receptors; all require F-actin recruitment (beneath tethered particles) and re-arrangement to promote engulfment; these processes are controlled by Rho family GTPases.

- **Exocytosis** (*and* **endocytosis**): organize the subcellular distribution of membrane-associated molecules, such as receptors, cell adhesion molecules, and cytoskeletal regulators. Goal: control signaling to the cell's external environments, and intracellularly as well. Exocytosis of trophic factors and extracellular proteinases act on surrounding microenvironments to affect cognate changes. Exocytic membrane fusion is mediated by an assembly of three *SNARE-family proteins*: 1) vesicle-associated membrane proteins (on vesicle membrane); 2) soluble N-ethylmaleimide-sensitive factor attachment proteins; and by 3) syntaxins (inner surface of target plasma membrane).
- **Endocytosis**: internalization of material via endocytosis may be receptor (e.g., clathrin) mediated or occur through formation of caveolae (i.e., membrane invaginations of the plasma membrane). These processes require unique structural and signalling machinery. Glycosphingolipids (GSL) are selectively internalized via caveolae; a selectivity which may occur because GSLs are involved in the formation of microdomains (i.e., *lipid rafts*). Clathrin-independent uptake mechanisms exist, via rhoA-dependent endocytosis of the interleukin 2 receptor ß subunit (IL-2Rß), and cdc42-regulated endocytosis of GPI-anchored proteins and fluid phase markers.
- **MHC class II-dependent antigen presentation**: processing of *internalized* exogenous antigens involves their binding to MHC class II molecules within endo-/lyso-somal compartments of antigen-presenting cells. In contrast, *cytoplasmic* autoantigens are degraded by the proteasome and other enzymes in the cytosol; then translocated to endo-/lyso-somal compartments for interaction with MHC class II molecules. These processes implicate roles for lysosome-associated membrane protein-2a (LAMP2a) and heat-shock cognate protein 70 (HSP70).

- **Suggested readings:**

*Cheng ZJ, Singh RD, Marks DL, Pagano RE. 2006. Membrane microdomains, caveolae, and caveolar endocytosis of sphingolipids. Mol Membr Biol. 23(1):101-10.*

*Ekyalongo RC, Nakayama H, Kina K, Kaga N, Iwabuchi K. 2015. Organization and functions* of *glycolipid-enriched microdomains in phagocytes. Biochim Biophys Acta. 1851(1):90-7.*

**Box 1.2. Animal models of LSD**

There are several animal models of disease, including those identified in large animals (such as cats, sheep and dogs) and mice; the latter generated through the application of recombinant genetic techniques.

Investigations involving animal models have provided considerable insights regarding pathophysiologic changes, with certain stipulations. Mouse models with mutations of the cognate gene often display evidence of tissue storage; however, the associated manifestations may not necessarily mimic the human condition. For instance, MLD (*Arsa* knockout) mice display a milder phenotype, with impaired coordination and deafness. Demyelination is absent and the ultrastructure of the myelin sheath is preserved, consistent with the lesser sulfatide storage observed in these affected mice. Interestingly, transgenic *Arsa* knockout mice overexpressing the enzymes of galactosphingolipid biosynthesis (as a means of increasing substrate storage) exhibit sulfatide accumulation not only in myelin-forming cells, but also in neurons. These mice develop severe neurological symptomatology, as observed in the human disease.

In contrast the *twitcher* (galactocerebrosidase-deficient) mouse represents an authentic human model of Krabbe disease. Interestingly, in a different mouse model of a late-onset, chronic form of Krabbe disease (generated by inactivating saposin A, the essential activator of galactocerebrosidase) pregnancy greatly improved neurological symptoms (compared to affected females that do not experience pregnancy, nor affected males). Demyelination with infiltration of globoid cells largely disappeared, and there was evidence of down-regulation of immune-related gene expression (MCP-1, TNF$\alpha$) in the brain. Additionally, there was increased expression of the estrogen receptors (ER$\alpha$ and ER$\beta$) on the globoid cells, activated astrocytes and microglia in demyelinating areas. In parallel experiments, pathology was also vastly improved in affected mice implanted with time-release 17 $\beta$-estradiol pellets (to simulate pregnancy). The clinical significance of these observations is not certain, but potentially points to a therapeutic avenue worth exploring.

*HexA*-deficient mice also do not develop neurological symptoms. In this case, murine sialidase enables conversion of $G_{M2}$ to $G_{A2}$ (degraded by *HexB*). On the other hand, *HexB-deficient* mice mimic human $G_{M2}$-gangliosidoses. Studies have shown neuroinflammatory changes (evident as microglial and astrocyte activation) are a concomitant pathologic event.

Animal models, primarily affected mice, have been used in pre-clinical 'proof of concept' studies to demonstrate administration of a putative therapeutic agent enabled substrate clearance; and were also valuable in examination of drug dose-response relationships. In α-glucosidase-deficient (Pompe disease) quails, administration of the recombinant enzyme (rhGAA) was shown to improve muscle strength, based on the flip test which looked at the ability of affected quails to right themselves from the supine position.

Animal models have also been used to explore delivery of the experimental therapeutic agents; particularly the means required to overcome the blood brain barrier. As most LSDs have primary CNS involvement, prevention of disease progression, stabilization or reversal of pathology within the brain will be essential. Concerns have been raised that such studies in mice may not be suitable for these purposes, given the small brain size and simplicity in brain architecture. Mouse brains typically weigh 0.5 gram, whereas the brain of a typical 5-year-old child is 450 grams. Moreover, mice have lissencephalic brains lacking gyri and sulci. Thus, more recently investigational studies have involved dogs and sheep, which have gyrencephalic brains weighing about 70 and 175 grams, respectively. In addition, larger animals have a longer span enabling extended periods of observation.

**Suggested readings:**

*Matsuda J, Vanier MT, Saito Y, Suzuki K, Suzuki K. 2001. Dramatic phenotypic improvement during pregnancy in a genetic leukodystrophy: estrogen appears to be a critical factor. Hum Mol Genet. 10(23):2709-15.*

*Suzuki K, Ezoe T, Tohyama J, Matsuda J, Vanier MT, Suzuki K. 2003. Are animal models useful for understanding the pathophysiology of lysosomal storage disease? Acta Paediatr Suppl. 92(443):54-62;*

*Zigdon H, Meshcheriakova A, Futerman AH. 2014. From sheep to mice to cells: tools for the study of the sphingolipidoses. Biochim Biophys Acta. 1841(8):1189-99.*

## Box 1.3. Autophagy, mTORC1, Lysosomal nutrient sensing (LyNUS) apparatus and the activation of autophagosome-lysosome related genes

*(see Figures 1.6 and 1.7)*

As a site for the digestion of complex macromolecules, lysosomes provide a source of basic building blocks that feed the biosynthetic requirements of the cell. This process is regulated through mTORC1 signalling and mediated by the nuclear translocation of TFEB, which - in turn - leads to transcription of autophagy- and lysosome-related genes. The coordinated expression of these gene sets is made possible by the binding of TFEB to an E-box like response element found within the promoters of relevant proteins. [Note: *TFEB is maintained in an 'off' state by dynamic recruitment to the cytoplasmic surface of lysosomes via Rag GTPase mediated-interaction with 14-3-3 chaperone protein.*]

The mammalian target of rapamycin (mTOR) is a conserved serine/threonine kinase and a member of the phosphatidylinositol 3-kinase (PI3K) pathway; comprising two different protein complexes: mTORC1 and mTORC2.

mTORCs are involved with several cellular responses and serve as links for cross-talk between several pathways (e.g., AMP-Kinase-TSC2 dependent mechanisms). mTORC1 specific partners include Raptor (regulatory-associated protein of mammalian target of rapamycin) and PRAS40 (proline-rich Akt substrate 40 kDa) (*Figure 1.6*). In its inactive state, mTORC1 is found on the lysosomal membrane in complex with Rag GTPases; which brings it into proximity with Rheb. [Rag GTPases are tethered to the surface of lysosomes by a membrane-anchored complex, Ragulator; made up of the Late endo-/lyso-somal adaptor, MAP-Kinase and mTOR activator 1-5. The function of Ragulator is dependent on its interaction with V-ATPase; which serves a role in detection of amino acid concentration within the lysosome, besides the acidification of the lysosome microenvironment.]

mTORC1 signalling may also be dependent in part on SLC38A9, an arginine and/or glutamine transporter on the lysosomal membrane, which co-purifies with Ragulator and Rag GTPase.

**Suggested readings:**

*Settembre C, Ballabio A. 2014. Lysosomal adaptation: how the lysosome responds to external cues. Cold Spring Harb Perspect Biol. 6(6).*

*Settembre C, Di Malta C, Polito VA, Garcia Arencibia M, Vetrini F, Erdin S, Erdin SU, Huynh T, Medina D, Colella P, Sardiello M, Rubinsztein DC, Ballabio A. 2011. TFEB links autophagy to lysosomal biogenesis. Science. 332(6036):1429-33.*

*Settembre C, Medina DL. 2015. TFEB and the CLEAR network. Methods Cell Biol. 126:45-62.*

**Box 1.4. Targeting of nascent proteins to the lysosome**

The majority of lysosomal hydrolases are tagged with phosphorylated mannose residues and gain access to the lysosome via the cation-independent mannose-6-phosphate (M6P) receptor. M6P modification is achieved by the addition of GlcNAc-1-phosphate to mannose residues and the subsequent removal of GlcNAc by an uncovering enzyme (UCE) (*Figure 1.3*). Studies have indicated dynamin plays an important role in the molecular machinery behind the recycling of the M6P receptor from endo-/lyso-somes to the *trans*-Golgi network, and may also be required for the final scission of vesicles budding from endosome tubules. Mice deficient in the formation of M6P residues exhibit significant loss of cathepsin proteases in B cells, leading to lysosomal dysfunction with accumulation of storage material, impaired antigen processing and presentation, and subsequent defects in B cell maturation and antibody production. The endosome to trans-Golgi transport, recycling and reuse of several proteins including the M6P receptor is mediated by VPS35, a component of the retromer complex.

Alternative processes of lysosomal targeting are mediated by other receptors, including lysosomal integral membrane *protein-2* (LIMP-2) and sortilin. LIMP-2 is involved in the delivery of β–glucosidase to the lysosome. Sortilin (100 kDa) appears to be a multifunctional receptor capable of binding several different ligands, including neurotensin and receptor-associated protein (RAP), and of targeting several proteins to the lysosome, including sphingolipid activator proteins (prosaposin and $G_{M2}$-activator protein), acid sphingomyelinase and cathepsins D and H.

**Suggested readings:**

*Braulke T, Bonifacino JS. 2009. Sorting of lysosomal proteins. Biochim Biophys Acta. 1793(4):605-14.*

*Canuel M, Korkidakis A, Konnyu K, Morales CR. 2008. Sortilin mediates the lysosomal targeting of cathepsins D and H. Biochem Biophys Res Commun. 373(2):292-7.*

*Coutinho MF, Prata MJ, Alves S. 2012. Mannose-6-phosphate pathway: a review on its role in lysosomal function and dysfunction. Mol Genet 105(4):542-50.*

*Coutinho MF, Prata MJ, Alves S. 2012. A shortcut to the lysosome: the mannose-6-phosphate-independent pathway. Mol Genet Metab. 107(3):257-66.*

*Lin SX, Mallet WG, Huang AY, Maxfield FR. 2004. Endocytosed cation-independent mannose 6-phosphate receptor traffics via the endocytic recycling compartment en route to the trans-Golgi network and a subpopulation of late endosomes. Mol Biol Cell. 15(2):721-33.*

*Otomo T, Schweizer M, Kollmann K, Schumacher V, Muschol N, Tolosa E, Mittrücker HW, Braulke T. Mannose 6 phosphorylation of lysosomal enzymes controls B cell functions. J Cell Biol. 2015 Jan 19;208(2):171-80.*

# References

[1] Medina DL, Fraldi A, Bouche V, Annunziata F, Mansueto G, Spampanato C, Puri C, Pignata A, Martina JA, Sardiello M, Palmieri M, Polishchuk R, Puertollano R, Ballabio A. 2011. Transcriptional activation of lysosomal exocytosis promotes cellular clearance. *Dev Cell.* 21(3):421-30.

[2] Eskelinen EL, Tanaka Y, Saftig P. 2003. At the acidic edge: emerging functions for lysosomal membrane proteins. *Trends Cell Biol.* 13(3): 137-45.

[3] Luzio JP, Hackmann Y, Dieckmann NM, Griffiths GM. 2014. The biogenesis of lysosomes and lysosome-related organelles. *Cold Spring Harb Perspect Biol.* 6(9):a016840.

[4] Marks MS, Heijnen HF, Raposo G. 2013. Lysosome-related organelles: unusual compartments become mainstream. *Curr Opin Cell Biol.* 25(4):495-505.

[5] Odorizzi G. 2015. Membrane manipulations by the ESCRT machinery. F1000Res. 4(F1000 Faculty Rev):516.

[6] Jiang S, Li Y, Zhang X, Bu G, Xu H, Zhang YW. 2014. Trafficking regulation of proteins in Alzheimer's disease. *Mol Neurodegener.* 9:6.

[7] Wilke S, Krausze J, Büssow K. 2012. Crystal structure of the conserved domain of the DC lysosomal associated membrane protein: implications for the lysosomal glycocalyx. *BMC Biol.* 10:62.

[8] Endo Y, Furuta A, Nishino I. 2015. Danon disease: a phenotypic expression of LAMP-2 deficiency. *Acta Neuropathol.* 129(3):391-8.

[9] Amaya C, Fader CM, Colombo MI. 2015. Autophagy and proteins involved in vesicular trafficking. *FEBS Lett.* 589(22):3343-53.

[10] Tanaka Y, Chambers JK, Matsuwaki T, Yamanouchi K, Nishihara M. 2014. Possible involvement of lysosomal dysfunction in pathological changes of the brain in aged progranulin-deficient mice. *Acta Neuropathol Commun.* 2:78.

[11] Thomas M, Alegre-Abarrategui J, Wade-Martins R. 2013. RNA dysfunction and aggrephagy at the centre of an amyotrophic lateral sclerosis/frontotemporal dementia disease continuum. *Brain.* 136 (Pt 5):1345-60.

[12] Coutinho MF, Prata MJ, Alves S. 2012. Mannose-6-phosphate pathway: a review on its role in lysosomal function and dysfunction. *Mol Genet Metab.* 105(4):542-50.

[13] Dierks T, Schlotawa L, Frese MA, Radhakrishnan K, von Figura K, Schmidt B. 2009. Molecular basis of multiple sulfatase deficiency, mucolipidosis II/III and Niemann-Pick C1 disease - Lysosomal storage disorders caused by defects of non-lysosomal proteins. *Biochim. Biophys.* 1793(4):710-25.

[14] Coutinho MF, Prata MJ, Alves S. 2012. A shortcut to the lysosome: the mannose-6-phosphate-independent pathway. *Mol Genet Metab.* 107(3):257-66.

[15] Carlo AS, Nykjaer A, Willnow TE. 2014. Sorting receptor sortilin-a culprit in cardiovascular and neurological diseases. *J Mol Med* (Berl). 92(9):905-11.

[16] Cotter K, Stransky L, McGuire C, Forgac M. 2015. Recent Insights into the Structure, Regulation, and Function of the V-ATPases. *Trends Biochem Sci.* 40(10):611-22.

[17] Hu Y, Carraro-Lacroix LR, Wang A, Owen C, Bajenova E, Corey PN, Brumell JH, Voronov I. 2015. Lysosomal pH Plays a Key Role in Regulation of mTOR Activity in Osteoclasts. *J Cell Biochem.*

[18] Lee JH, McBrayer MK, Wolfe DM, Haslett LJ, Kumar A, Sato Y, Lie PP, Mohan P, Coffey EE, Kompella U, Mitchell CH, Lloyd-Evans E, Nixon RA. 2015. Presenilin 1 Maintains Lysosomal $Ca^{2+}$ Homeostasis via TRPML1 by Regulating vATPase-Mediated Lysosome Acidification. *Cell Rep.* 12(9):1430-44.

[19] Ramachandran N, Munteanu I, Wang P, Ruggieri A, Rilstone JJ, Israelian N, Naranian T, Paroutis P, Guo R, Ren ZP, Nishino I, Chabrol B, Pellissier JF, Minetti C, Udd B, Fardeau M, Tailor CS, Mahuran DJ, Kissel JT, Kalimo H, Levy N, Manolson MF, Ackerley CA, Minassian BA. 2013. VMA21 deficiency prevents vacuolar ATPase assembly and causes autophagic vacuolar myopathy. *Acta Neuropathol.* 125(3): 439-57.

[20] Settembre C, Medina DL. 2015. TFEB and the CLEAR network. *Methods Cell Biol.* 126:45-62.

[21] Martina JA, Diab HI, Lishu L, Jeong-A L, Patange S, Raben N, Puertollano R. 2014. The nutrient-responsive transcription factor TFE3 promotes autophagy, lysosomal biogenesis, and clearance of cellular debris. *Sci Signal.* 7(309):ra9.

[22] Settembre C, Fraldi A, Medina DL, Ballabio A. 2013. Signals from the lysosome: a control centre for cellular clearance and energy metabolism. *Nat Rev Mol Cell Biol.* 14(5):283-96.

[23] Jin M, Klionsky DJ. 2015. The amino acid transporter SLC38A9 regulates MTORC1 and autophagy. *Autophagy.* 11(10):1709-10.

[24] Patel S, Docampo R. 2010. Acidic calcium stores open for business: expanding the potential for intracellular $Ca^{2+}$ signalling. *Trends Cell Biol.* 20(5):277-86.

[25] Marchant JS, Patel S. 2015. Two-pore channels at the intersection of endolysosomal membrane traffic. *Biochem Soc Trans.* 43(3):434-41.

[26] Hui L, Geiger NH, Bloor-Young D, Churchill GC, Geiger JD, Chen X. 2015. Release of calcium from endolysosomes increases calcium influx through N-type calcium channels: Evidence for acidic store-operated calcium entry in neurons. *Cell Calcium.*

[27] Medina DL, Di Paola S, Peluso I, Armani A, De Stefani D, Venditti R, Montefusco S, Scotto-Rosato A, Prezioso C, Forrester A, Settembre C, Wang W, Gao Q, Xu H, Sandri M, Rizzuto R, De Matteis MA, Ballabio A. 2015. Lysosomal calcium signalling regulates autophagy through calcineurin and TFEB. *Nat Cell Biol.* 17(3):288-99.

[28] Cheng X, Zhang X, Yu L, Xu H. 2015. Calcium signalling in membrane repair. *Semin Cell Dev Biol.*

[29] Blazek AD, Paleo BJ, Weisleder N. 2015. Plasma Membrane Repair: A Central Process for Maintaining Cellular Homeostasis. *Physiology* (Bethesda). 30(6):438-48.

[30] Kovtun O, Tillu VA, Ariotti N, Parton RG, Collins BM. 2015. Cavin family proteins and the assembly of caveolae. *J Cell Sci.* 128(7): 1269-78.

[31] Duraes FV, Niven J, Dubrot J, Hugues S, Gannagé M. 2015. Macroautophagy in Endogenous Processing of Self- and Pathogen-Derived Antigens for MHC Class II Presentation. *Front Immunol.* 6:459.

[32] Michelet X, Garg S, Wolf BJ, Tuli A, Ricciardi-Castagnoli P, Brenner MB. 2015. MHC class II presentation is controlled by the lysosomal small GTPase, Arl8b. *J Immunol.* 194(5):2079-88.

[33] Ohkouchi S, Shibata M, Sasaki M, Koike M, Safig P, Peters C, Nagata S, Uchiyama Y. 2013. Biogenesis and proteolytic processing of lysosomal DNase II. *PLoS One*. 8(3):e59148.

[34] Oka T, Hikoso S, Yamaguchi O, Taneike M, Takeda T, Tamai T, Oyabu J, Murakawa T, Nakayama H, Nishida K, Akira S, Yamamoto A, Komuro I, Otsu K. 2012. Mitochondrial DNA that escapes from autophagy causes inflammation and heart failure. *Nature*. 485(7397): 251-5.

*Chapter 2*

# Pathobiology

Lysosomal storage diseases are monogenic disorders, although multiple mutations have been described for the various individual conditions which can lead to complete loss of function (or some residual activity) of the cognate protein. The nature of the underlying gene defect partly explains the variability seen in age at onset, rate of disease progression and overall severity. Null alleles lead to severe, early onset phenotypes; whilst missense mutations (associated with residual protein activity) tend to cause an attenuated disease, which is not to say that burden on physical and functional well-being is minimal. Other factors that modify disease expression have not been fully clarified (*see* Box 2.1). Furthermore, the mechanistic links between substrate storage and organ damage remains to be delineated, but likely involves several interrelated disease pathways.

It is increasingly clear that lysosomes have several and more complex functions than simply being the end-point on a degradative track. While intralysosomal accumulation of incompletely metabolized substrates represents the initial insult to cells (deficient in hydrolytic capacity or that harbor a defect in substrate transport), ultimately impairment of cellular homeostasis results from a combination of disease mechanisms (Figure 2.1). There has been increasing interest in the role of lysosomal dysfunction associated with certain LSDs, as possibly contributing to the development of conditions seen in elderly populations (Table 2.1).

The various roles normally served by the different substrates are incompletely understood, but likely manifold. For instance, glycosaminoglycans (GAG) are believed to be engaged in the trafficking of molecules through the endosomal network, and maintenance of the steady state levels of intra- and extra-cellular oligosaccharides and proteoglycans, the activity of lysosomal enzymes, and regulation of GAG-dependent inhibitors (serpins or serine proteinase inhibitors and cathepsins) [1]. Cysteine cathepsins are a group of enzymes normally found in endolysosomes where they are primarily involved in intracellular protein turnover, but also have a critical role in MHC II-mediated antigen processing and presentation. Investigations of cathepsin activities have revealed glycosaminoglycans facilitate the autocatalytic activation of cathepsins, including at neutral pH in the extracellular matrix, and critically modulate their activities (such as in the case of the collagenolytic activity of cathepsin K) [2]. More recently, a system biology approach revealed several reactions potentially impaired in the mucopolysaccharidoses (i.e., defects of GAG metabolism), including those mainly involved in cellular respiration, mitochondrial processes, amino acid and lipid metabolism, and ion exchange [3].

Certain molecules generated from metabolism within the lysosome, such as ceramide and sphingosine and their phosphorylated counterparts, are recognized as "bioactive sphingolipids"; molecules that modulate membrane integrity, the activity of enzymes, or act as ligands of G protein-coupled receptors [4]. The importance of these substrates is underscored by the fact that sphingomyelin (SM) in the brain accounts for about 15% of the total phospholipids, while galactocerebrosides for approximately 15% of total human brain lipids (which, altogether amounts to about half of the brain's dry weight). Sphingomyelin is the primary substrate which accumulates in Niemann-Pick disease types A/B; whereas galactocerebrosides is the substrate not fully catabolized by patients with Krabbe disease (β-galactocerebrosidase deficiency).

**Table 2.1. LSDs and associated condition**

| Disorder | Associated conditions |
|---|---|
| Gaucher disease | Parkinsonism/Lewy body formation |
| Niemann-Pick disease type C, MPS-IIIB | Alzheimer disease |
| CLN11 disease (progranulin mutation) | Frontotemporal lobar dementia with TDP-43 inclusions |
| MPS-IIIA (SGSH mutations) | Adult-onset NCL |

Ceramide is generated by (1) *de novo* synthesis (catalyzed by serine palmitoyl transferase, SPTLC), (2) the removal of the head group of more complex sphingolipids (e.g., sphingomyelin), or (3) via the sphingosine salvage pathway. Acid sphingomyelinase is mainly localized to the lumen of late endosomes/lysosomes, where it degrades endocytosed SM on intraluminal vesicles.

Deficiency of acid sphingomyelinase is the cause of Niemann-Pick disease type A/B (*see* Figure 2.2, illustrating associated defects in sequential degradation of sphingolipids *and* Box 2.2). Reduced *de novo* sphingolipid synthesis (resulting from *SPTLC* mutations) is associated with hereditary sensory and autonomic neuropathy type I (HSAN-I), an inherited autosomal dominant neurological disease characterized by loss of pain and temperature sensation and damaged autonomic functions (manifested by altered sweating and light headedness).

Recently, several defects in the synthesis of certain sphingolipids that eventually end up as lysosomal substrates have been described (*see* Figure 2.3 *and* Box 2.3); their elucidation may contribute to a fuller understanding of the physiologic roles of the relevant substrates, and the consequences of a disturbance in their metabolism.

A disruption in metabolism can lead to a tipping point (i.e., breached threshold), following which compensatory or adoptive measures ultimately become deleterious in the stimulating presence of excess substrates. Increasingly, there is appreciation of shared disease pathways, across a spectrum of etiologies. Changes in the concentration or activity of several analytes are detectable in various LSDs, and there is an active interest in the potential usefulness of intermediary metabolites as biomarkers and indicators of disease activity (*see* Box 2.4).

It should be noted that although distinct deficiencies of lysosomal hydrolases can lead to the accumulation of the cognate enzyme's primary substrate, other substances can be accrued; interestingly, these secondary substrates may not be found in the same subcellular compartment [5]. For instance, in Sanfilippo syndrome (MPS-III), the primary defect is in heparan sulfate catabolism. The accumulation of dermatan sulfate (DS) as a secondary metabolite has been observed. Investigations indicate heparan sulfate and heparin can inhibit iduronate 2-sulfatase (enzyme deficient in MPS-II), and this is the most likely explanation for DS build up [6].

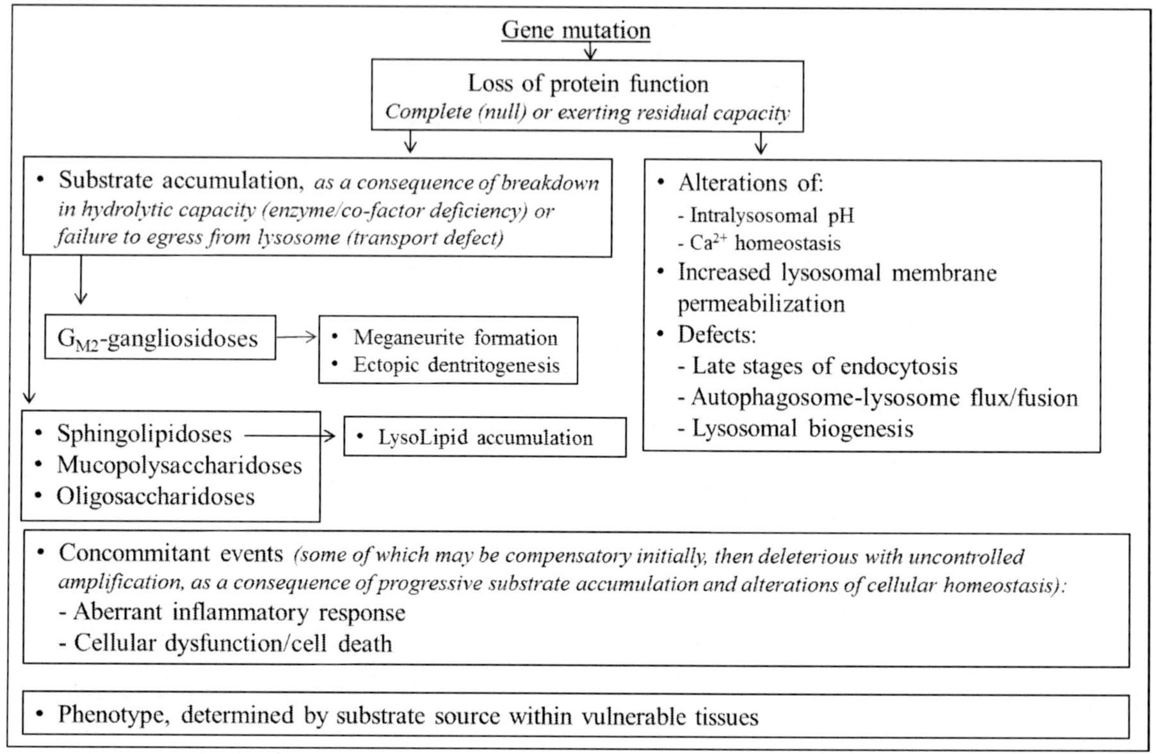


Figure 2.1. Lysosomal dysfunction and interlocking events.

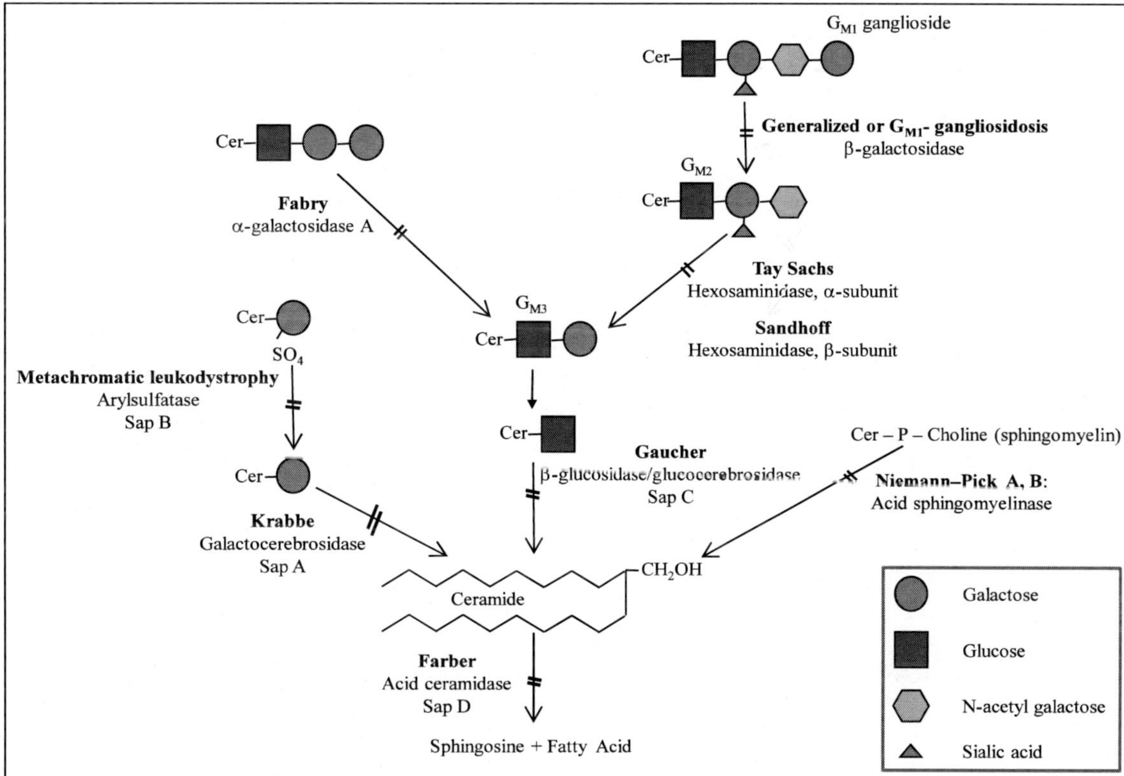


Figure 2.2. Sphingolipid catabolism and associated disorders. The hydrolysis of certain glycosphingolipids requires a co-factor, such as the saposins; *see* Box 2.2.

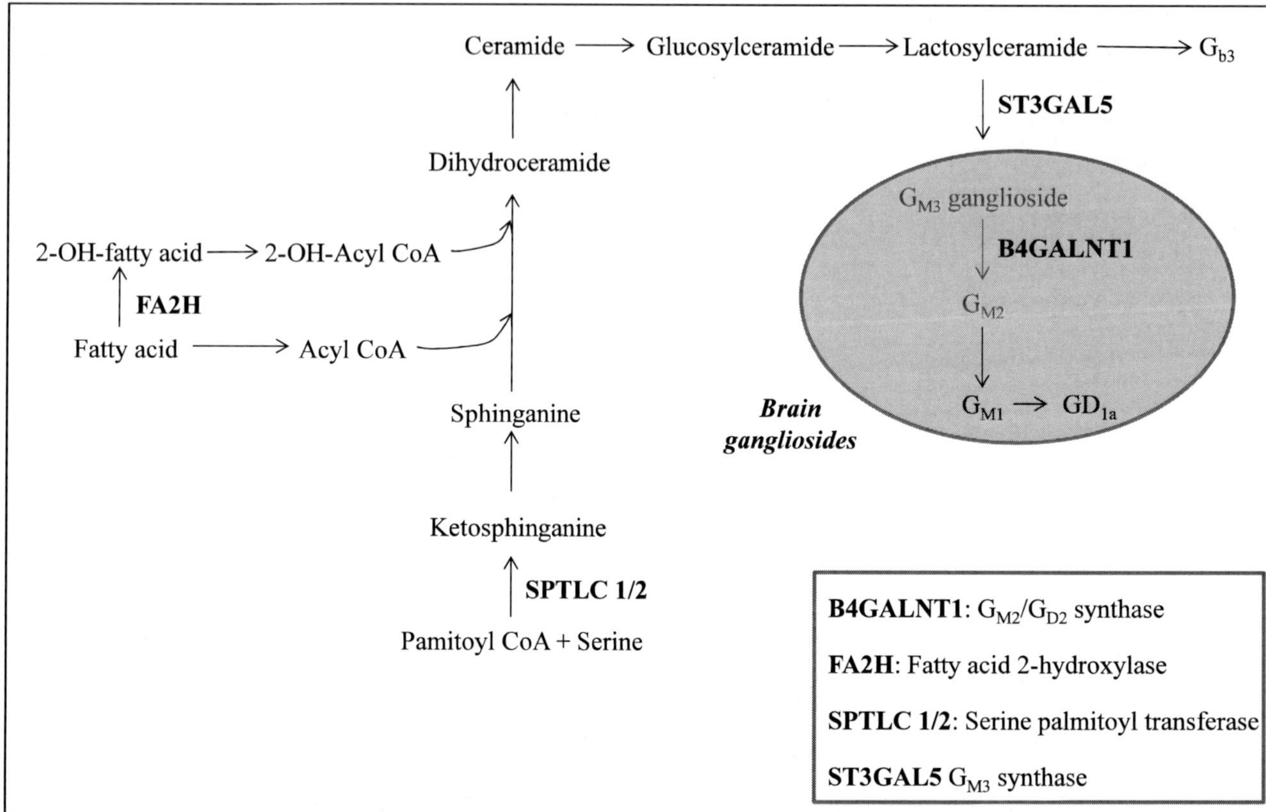


Figure 2.3. Sphingolipid synthesis and associated disorders (*see* Box 2.3).

Increased energy expenditure for the synthesis of substrates trapped within lysosomes has been proposed as furthering the disease process, with energy imbalance as a basis for the decreased adiposity described in patients with certain LSDs and in corresponding animal models [7]. In a study involving the MPS-I mouse model, metabolite analysis identified deficiencies in simple sugars, nucleotides, and lipids in the liver; findings which are suggestive of a disturbance in intermediary metabolism, perhaps linked with increased autophagy (*which can be triggered by a "fasting" state*) [8].

Insights regarding pathological mechanisms for most LSDs have been gained primarily from investigations of various animal models of disease. In these models, tissue samples can be obtained and analyzed prior to onset of disease manifestations and thereafter; which almost is impossible to achieve with humans, given the all too common delay in clinical diagnosis. Nevertheless, valuable insights have also been derived from examination of tissues from affected human subjects, mainly fibroblasts. In the latter case, it is not certain whether observations are generalizable to other cell types, particularly neurons. More recently, manipulation of patient derived-inducible pluripotent stem cells (iPSCs) and their differentiation to specific cell types of interest have become a major source of complementary information regarding pathogenesis.

## a. Morphological Findings

Unlike other inborn errors of metabolism (i.e., defects of amino and organic acid metabolism) which can be associated with acute decompensation due to 'intoxication,' most patients with an LSD (including those with ultimate neuropathic involvement) are clinically normal at birth, and growth and developmental pattern in the first weeks of life is often uneventful. Exceptions to these are severe, early onset presentations, characterized by non-immune *hydrops fetalis* [9]. Also, patients with I-cell disease (mucolipidosis II) and early infantile $G_{M1}$-gangliosidosis may show dysmorphic features at birth or in the early months of life. Dysmorphic features are apparent in the second six months of life in patients with Hurler syndrome (MPS-I), but may not be picked up by those without prior experience. In these cases, lateral spine and hand X-rays may show evidence of skeletal dysplasia (*dysostosis multiplex*). Obviously, family history and knowledge of *a priori* risk may enable diagnostic confirmation prenatally or at birth in relevant circumstances.

The accumulation of incompletely metabolized material is the hallmark of LSDs. In conditions associated with $G_{M2}$-ganglioside accumulation, affected neurons are transformed into meganeurites and display ectopic dendrites [10]. Normally, a burst of neurite outgrowth occurs during early cortical development, and morphologically mature pyramidal neurons do not sprout additional primary dendrites thereafter. $G_{M2}$-ganglioside has been proposed as a functional component of glycosphingolipid-enriched microdomains (i.e., lipid rafts found in the plasmalemma, *see* Box 2.5); promoting dendritic initiation through modulation of specific membrane proteins and/or their associated second messenger cascades. Storage of $G_{M2}$-ganglioside may lead to aberrant propagation of this process, which is limited to cortical pyramidal neurons and multipolar neurons in the claustrum and amygdala.

Overexpression of GluR2 subunit in cultured neurons has been shown to induce ectopic dendritic spine formation, implicating α-amino-3-hydroxy-5-methylisoxazole-propionic acid (AMPA) receptor expression in the process of dendritic and synaptic plasticity [11]. Recent data suggest hippocampal neurons N-cadherin and GluR2 form a synaptic complex that stimulates presynaptic development and function, as well as promoting dendritic spine formation [12]. Interestingly, conditional inactivation of chemokine (C-X-C motif) receptor 4 (*Cxcr4*[10]) in the central nervous system of mice has been shown to lead to defects in Purkinje cell[11] dendritogenesis and axonal projection *in vivo* but not in cell culture [13]. The relationship of this phenomenon to $G_{M2}$-ganglioside metabolism is not certain, and could well be a distinct process.

In sialidosis (neuraminidase deficiency), examination of the cerebellar vermis obtained from an affected individual has revealed dysplastic features: *viz.*, abnormal layering of Purkinje cells, thinning and rarefaction of the granule cell layer, incomplete formation of synapse, and disordered proliferation of Bergmann's glia [14]. These observations were deemed a developmental abnormality, and possibly related to abnormal signalling. Studies in the corresponding mouse model showed deficiency of lysosomal

---

[10] CXCR4 is a receptor of the chemokine CXCL12; it is expressed in spinal cord radial glia and has been shown to control the integrity of radial glial scaffold in developing spinal cord. CXCL12, more commonly referred to as stromal-derived factor-1 (SDF-1), acts as a chemoattractant for a variety of adult stem cells including mesenchymal stem cells, hematopoietic stem cells, neural progenitor cells, and endothelial progenitor cells.

[11] Purkinje cells are a class of GABAergic neurons located in the cerebellum; named after their discoverer, the Czech anatomist Jan Evangelista Purkyně (1787-1869).

sialidase (neuraminidase) led to the spontaneous occurrence of an Alzheimer disease-like amyloidogenic process [15].

Examination of brains from two different mouse models of neuronal ceroid lipofuscinosis (NCL) has revealed progressive breakdown of axons and synapses. Synaptic pathology was evident in the thalamus and cortex of these mice, but occurred much earlier within the thalamus. Quantitative comparisons of expression levels for a subset of proteins previously implicated in regulation of axonal and synaptic vulnerability revealed changes in proteins involved with synaptic function/stability and cell-cycle regulation in both affected mice strains. These changes were evident at pre/early-symptomatic stages, occurring in advance of morphologically detectable synaptic or axonal pathology with regional selectivity occurring first within the thalamus and only later in the cortex [16]. Analyses of gene expression patterns in other LSDs, prior to onset of symptoms may shed light on potentially shared early events that can be targets for therapy.

Examination of brain neurons from MPS-IIIA and –IIIB (Sanfilippo syndrome[12]) mice revealed over-expression of GM130 protein (a Golgi matrix protein) and alterations of Golgi ribbon architecture, enhanced proliferation and outgrowth of neurites and alteration of neural cell migration [17]. Separate studies in the MPS-IIIB mouse model have shown that the build-up of heparin sulfate (HS) oligosaccharides led to an activation of synaptophysin degradation by the proteasome, with consequences on synaptic vesicle components [18]. Alterations in GM130-mediated control of vesicle trafficking occurred, which affected Golgi biogenesis and gave rise to a dead-end storage compartment. Together, these findings likely account for neuron dysfunction and death in these conditions, and perhaps other MPS disorders with HS storage.

Of further relevance to the mucopolysaccharidoses, it has been shown that exposure of wild-type neural cells to exogenous soluble HS fragments (of at least eight saccharides) activated integrin-based focal adhesions (FAs), which are vital to attachment of cells to the extracellular matrix. FAs were found to be constitutively activated in MPS-IIIB astrocytes and neural stem cells, a phenomenon corrected by clearance of undigested saccharides, following

[12] Sanfilippo syndrome refers to one of five autosomal recessive neurodegenerative lysosomal storage disorders (MPS IIIA to MPS IIIE) whose symptoms are caused by the deficiency of enzymes involved exclusively in heparan sulfate degradation. Clinical features include mental retardation and hyperactivity, typically commencing during childhood. Bone involvement is not as prominent, as encountered in the other MPS syndromes.

provision of the missing exoglycanase [19]. Defective cell polarisation and oriented migration in response to focal extracellular stimuli in affected cells suggest there may be improper sensing of the environment. Brain imaging, with assessment of gray matter volume and tractography, may be useful in mapping changes within brains of affected individuals, which may prove to correlate with developmental outcomes.

Examination of the brain of the MPS-IIIB (α-*N*-acetylglucosaminidase deficiency) mouse model has revealed phosphorylated tau (P-tau) in the medial entorhinal cortex (MEC) [20]. Electron microscopy of neurons from the dentate gyrus (a part of the hippocampal formation receiving major input from the entorhinal cortex) showed cytoplasmic inclusions of paired helical filaments; i.e., P-tau aggregates characteristic of tauopathies[13]. There was elevation of glypican, and it has been proposed extralysosomal glypican is harmful to neurons, because its heparan sulfate branches could potentiate the formation of P-tau and beta amyloid aggregates, which would be toxic as well as difficult to degrade [21].

Glycogen synthase kinase-3 beta (GSK-3β) activity can be induced by Aβ (the principal protein implicated in Alzheimer disease), promoting extensive phosphorylation of tau and cell death. Interestingly, P-tau inclusions were reduced in number when affected MPS-IIIB mice were administered LiCl, a specific inhibitor of GSK-3β [20].

Examination of neuronal ceroid lipofuscinosis (CLN3) patient-derived iPS cells revealed marked aberrations of the endo/lysosomal compartment, evidenced by large LAMP1-positive ring-like structures (detected by immunofluorescence) and cytoplasmic vacuolations (evident on electron micrographs) [21]. Also noted was an increase in the size of autophagic vacuoles. These observations were viewed as likely reflecting defects in lysosomal maturation, pH maintenance and/or in the fusion of lysosomes with autophagosomes[14].

---

[13] In the central nervous system, tau is the major microtubule-associated protein (MAP) of neurons, promoting assembly and stabilization of microtubules required for morphogenesis and axonal transport. Primary tauopathies are characterized by deposition of abnormal fibrils of tau in neuronal and glial cells, leading to neuronal death, brain atrophy and eventually dementia. In these conditions, a cascade of neuronal reactions, such as activation of glycogen synthase kinase-3β, mitogen-activated protein kinases, cell cycle re-entry and oxidative stress, lead to progressive neurodegeneration.

[14] Neuronal ceroid lipofuscinoses refers to a group of primarily childhood neurodegenerative disorders, currently associated with mutations in 13 genes; encoding proteins localized mostly in lysosomes (CLN1, CLN2, CLN3, CLN5, CLN7, CLN10, CLN12 and CLN13),

Limited brain autopsies on affected children with an LSD have not provided the types of information derived from an animal studies; perhaps, because human samples, if available, were obtained in the terminal stage of disease process. On the other hand, most of the above-described studies have been conducted in mice models, which need to be correlated with investigations of brains from large animal models (e.g., canine, ovine) to ascertain whether these observations are a factor in pathogenesis and their putative relevance to human subjects.

## b. Chronic Activation of the Innate Inflammatory Response

The inflammatory reaction is a normal physiologic response to harmful stimuli; but, it can also lead to destructive changes when chronically activated and unchecked. Aberrant inflammatory responses, which ultimately lead to cell death, are instrumental factors in the neurodegenerative process associated with certain LSDs.

Normally, glycolipid ligands for invariant NKT (iNKT) cells are loaded onto CD1d molecules in endo-/lyso-somes. Accumulation of glycosphingolipids (GSL) associated with certain LSDs has been hypothesized to influence lipid loading and/or antigen presentation, causing entrapment of endogenous ligand(s) within storage bodies or competition of the selecting ligand(s) by stored lipids for CD1d binding. These changes may be partly related to or influence alterations of plasma membrane lipid rafts.

Analyses of the iNKT cell compartment in LSD animal models that accumulate GSLs, glycosaminoglycans or both, revealed defective iNKT cell selection only in animals affected by multiple sulfatase deficiency[15], in which

the endoplasmic reticulum (CLN6 and CLN8), or in the cytosol associated with vesicular membranes (CLN4 and CLN14). CLN1 (palmitoyl protein thioesterase 1), CLN2 (tripeptidyl-peptidase 1), CLN5, CLN10 (cathepsin D), and CLN13 (cathepsin F), are lysosomal soluble proteins; others like CLN3, CLN7, and CLN12, have been proposed to be lysosomal transmembrane proteins.

[15] Multiple sulfatase deficiency is caused by a deficiency of the enzyme sulfatase modifying factor 1 (SUMF1); which is required for the catalytic activation of all eukaryotic sulfatases, in a post-translational modification step wherein a conserved cysteine within the active site is converted in the endoplasmic reticulum to a $C_\alpha$-formylglycine (*see* Figure 1.3). SUMF1 deficiency ablates the function of all sulfatases, and intralysosomal accumulation of various substrates.

a generalized aberrant T-cell development, rather than a pure iNKT defect, was present [22]. In another study, the percentages and frequency of iNKT cells were reduced in multiple mouse models of lysosomal GSL storage disease, irrespective of the specific genetic defect or lipid species stored [23]. The reduced numbers of iNKT cells resulted in the absence of cytokine production in response to α-galactosylceramide exposure, which is known to activate both human and mouse iNKT cells. This observation in one of the models examined, specifically *NPC1* null mice (with secondary GSL storage), was not confirmed; following examination of samples from human NPC patients (which revealed normal frequencies and function of iNKT cells) [24]. Thus, further studies are required to clarify the clinical significance of these varied observations.

Microglia and astrocytes are main components of the innate immune response within the CNS; with microglia engaged in detection of harmful/injurious agents, and astrocytes tied up with neurotrophic support and tissue homeostasis. Toll-like receptors (TLR) are expressed on the surface of several cell types, including microglia and astrocytes, and are involved with recognizing endogenous (damage-associated, DAMPs) or exogenous (pathogen-associated, PAMPs) molecular patterns that indicate tissue damage or the presence of foreign bodies (e.g., pathogens) [24]. Ligation of TLR results in cellular activation, phagocytosis and secretion of cytokines. Complement proteins also participate as receptors for DAMPs and PAMPs, in triggering neuroinflammation. Although initial activation of these process may represent attempts to address the underlying pathology, at some point a threshold is breached and there is amplification and subsequent activation of transduction pathways. The latter may include the production of inflammatory cytokines, reactive oxygen species and nitric oxide, with resultant deleterious consequences.

Activation of resident microglia and an influx of activated blood monocytes consequent to storage are deemed responsible for an inflammatory component of LSD brain disease. In its basal state, microglia exhibit a quiescent phenotype. Neurons play an integral role in maintaining this quiescent state, through the expression of membrane-bound ligands such as CD200 and CX3CL1, which function through cognate receptors on the surface of microglia [24]. Microglia can promote neuronal survival or exacerbate the disease process, depending on their activation profile. Activated microglia secretes cytokines that lead to activation of neighboring microglia, and can act on neurons to cause injury.

In MPS-IIIA and -IIIB, microglia and astrocytes from the corresponding mouse models have been shown to be activated through an interaction between TLR4 and the accumulated heparan sulfate oligosaccharides [25]. Although likely to be an aspect of the disease process, it is not the only element as inhibition of TLR4 signalling pathway in the case of the MPS-IIIB mouse model did not stop progression of the neurodegenerative course [26]. In these studies, oxidative stress was also a factor (*discussed in succeeding section*).

Separately, the role of TLR4 (and MD-2[16]) in the inflammatory process has been investigated in response to lipopolysaccharides (LPS, principal component of Gram-negative bacterial membrane) exposure. LPS recognition by TLR4 is usually followed by TLR4 dimerization on the cell surface, leading to the activation of downstream signalling pathways. Activated TLR4 is then transported from the plasma membrane to lysosomes, via endocytosis (which is dependent on clathrin-coated vesicles). Late endosome/lysosome-associated small Rab GTPase (Rab 7) regulates the translocation of TLR4 to lysosomes, where TLR4 is degraded; terminating LPS responses [27]. A disruption of this process may occur with certain LSDs, although there are no studies demonstrating any correlation between bacterial or viral infections and disease onset or exacerbation.

Examination of macrophages derived from peripheral monocytes obtained from patients with Gaucher disease[17] (GD) type 1 (homozygous for the p.N370S mutation) revealed the activation of the inflammasome[18] and increased secretion of interleukins (IL)-1β and IL-6 [28]. This phenomenon was shown to be a consequence of impaired autophagy (based on demonstration of elevated levels of the autophagic adaptor p62), which

---

[16] Myeloid differentiation factor 2 (MD2) is a small extracellular glycoprotein which serves as the main molecule for LPS recognition; it associates with TLR4, regulating its subsequent homotypic interaction. Recently, it has been hypothesized chronically low levels of circulating LPS (derived from the gut) may be associated with the development of metabolic diseases such as insulin resistance, type 2 diabetes, atherosclerosis and cardiovascular disease.

[17] Gaucher disease (GD) is an autosomal recessive LSD, caused by deficiency of the enzyme glucocererosidase (b-glucosidase) associated with consequent accumulation of the glycosphingolipid glucosylceramide (glucocerebrosaide). Cardinal manifestations in the non-neuronopathic subtype (1) include anemia, thrombocytopenia, heaptosplenoemagly and bone involvement. Patients with GD are at increased risk for cholelithiasis (gallstones), Parkinson disease and multiple myeloma.

[18] The inflammasome represents a multiprotein complex that plays an important role in innate immune sensing. Activation of inflammasomes leads to activation of caspase-1, and the maturation and secretion of the pro-inflammatory cytokines interleukin (IL)-1β and IL-18.

prevented the delivery of inflammasomes to autophagosomes. The link between lysosomal storage, impaired autophagy, and inflammation may have implications relevant to the increased risk for Parkinson disease seen in families segregating for mutations in the *GBA* gene (*see* Box 2.6). Treatment with the small-molecule β-glucosidase chaperone NCGC758 reversed these defects, inducing autophagy and reducing IL-1β secretion, which was deemed as pointing to a role for β-glucosidase deficiency in these processes [28].

Lipid storage in Gaucher disease is restricted to cells of monocyte/macrophage lineage. The increase in p62 (*as noted above*), also led to activation of p65-NF-kB in the nucleus and promoted the expression of inflammatory cytokines and secretion of IL-1β. These changes may be involved with the massive organomegaly, bone disease and increased susceptibility to certain malignancies seen in patients with GD [27]. Of potential relevance to the latter observation, a separate study revealed β-glucosylceramide 22:0 (βGL1-22) and glucosylsphingosine (LGL1), two major sphingolipids that accumulate in GD, can be recognized by a distinct subset of CD1d-restricted human and murine type II natural killer T (NKT) cells [29]. βGL1-22- and LGL1-specific NKT cells constitutively expressed a T-follicular helper (TFH) phenotype, and injection of these lipids into mice led to a downstream induction of germinal center B cells, hypergammaglobulinemia, and the production of antilipid antibodies. [TFH are fundamentally required for the generation of T cell-dependent B cell responses.] These obse4rvations may be relevant to increased risk for multiple myeloma among patients with GD.

## c. Defects of Autophagy

Defects of autophagy have been described in several LSDs; when associated with the accumulation of protein aggregates, this may be an added factor fostering neurodegeneration as post-mitotic cells such as neurons appear to be particularly vulvnerable to this type of situation. Changes in intracellular calcium homeostasis may represent an antecedent event (*discussed in the following section*).

Impairment of macroautophagy maturation has been found in juvenile CLN3 disease patients' fibroblasts, alongside with a 0.6 increase in lysosomal pH [30]. Similar abnormalities of autophagy have been found in iPS and neural progenitor cells derived from juvenile CLN3 disease iPS cells.

Cathepsin F has been implicated in the process of autophagy and proteasome[19]-mediated degradation. Mutations in *cathepsin F* (*CTSF*, *CLN13*) have been described in three families with adult-onset NCL associated with dementia and motor disturbances [31]. Confocal microscopy (in HEK 293T cells overexpressing either wild type or N-terminally truncated forms of cathepsin F) revealed that mutants displayed perinuclear inclusions, which were confirmed as p62-positive aggregates (a phagophore marker). It has been postulated the slow development of the disease may be caused by the function of cathepsin F being mildly affected, or that the loss of its function may be partly compensated and thus a long time is needed until the accumulated changes due to lysosomal/autophagic defects reaches a break-point, and disease symptoms begin to appear [32]. The same phenomenon may apply to other neurodegenerative processes encountered in the elderly population, such as Parkinson disease and Alzheimer disease, wherein slowly progressive lysosomal dysfunction (with resultant protein aggregation) has been postulated to occur; which may explain the prolonged period of latency.

A note on *mitophagy*, i.e., the selective elimination of damaged mitochondria through autophagy. The inability to clear damaged mitochondria may lead to dysregulated mitochondrial activity, which results in on-going generation of reactive oxygen species as a by-product of oxidative phosphorylation, and can cause damage to DNA and proteins.

Studies have shown that activation of Bcl-2-like protein 13 (Bcl2-L-13), localized on the outer mitochondrial membrane (OMM), induces mitochondrial fragmentation and mitophagy in mammalian cells [33]. Subsequent debris clearance occurs through the PINK1 (PTEN-induced putative kinase 1)/Parkin (PARK) pathway, mediated by autophagic adaptor proteins such as Fbxo7. [PINK1 is upstream of PARK function; when stabilized on the mitochondrial surface, it phosphorylates ubiquitin and recruits PARK from the cytosol, which then draws in multiple proteins onto the OMM. Mutations in *PINK1, PARK,* and *Fbxo7* have been associated with

[19] Ubiquitin-proteasome (UPS) pathway: Ubiquitin (Ub) is a signal for the degradation of polypeptides in the proteasome, and also involved with the recognition of cargoes destined for selective autophagy. Targets of UPS are proteins regulating a broad range of cellular processes including cell cycle progression, gene expression, the quality control of proteostasis and the response to geno- and proteo-toxic stresses. The proteasome exists as holo-enzymes composed of regulatory and core particles: a 19-subunit regulatory particle (RP) recognizes ubiquitin-tagged proteins, which removes ubiquitin and injects the target protein into the proteolytic chamber of the core particle (CP).

Parkinson disease.] Interestingly, the mechanism of failed PARK-mediated elimination of damaged mitochondria is not the same across several LSDs, in which such changes have been observed.

In multiple sulfatase deficiency, there is a significant reduction in PARK2 levels which leads to accumulation of morphologically aberrant mitochondria with reduced mitochondrial membrane potential ($\Delta\Psi_m$) and ATP production; as a consequence, apoptosis sets in [34]. In type II Gaucher disease, the level of PARK2 is unchanged; however, the ability of the dysfunctional mitochondria to recruit PARK2 is compromised [35]. In Pompe disease[20], PARK2 is increased in affected myotubes and to a greater extent in α-glucosidase (GAA) knock-out (KO) muscle; additionally, in the latter tissue levels of both PINK1 and PARK2 are increased in the mitochondrial fraction, which indicates that the translocation of PARK2 to damaged mitochondria and the subsequent ubiquitination of mitochondrial proteins are not impaired [36]. However, when the KO myotubes were infected with a virus expressing mCherry–GFP tag attached to the OMM localization signal of the FIS1[21] protein (residues 101 to 152), a significant number of damaged mitochondria remained in the cytosol, suggesting their inefficient clearance through mitophagy (attributed to incomplete autophagic flux).

Mitochondrial turnover may occur by additional-PINK1/PARK-independent-pathways, and defects of PINK1 and PARK function may impact mitochondrial regulation by mechanisms potentially separate from mitophagy These issues, and their relevance to LSDs needs further investigations.

[20] Pompe disease is an autosomal recessive LSD, caused by deficiency of the enzyme α-glucosidase associated with accumulation of glycogen, primarily in muscle tissue. The infantile onset form is characterized by cardiomyopathy and hypotonia in the first 3-6 months of life. There is a late-onset variant, wherein proximal muscle weakness and diaphragmatic weakness (leading to apnea) are prominent features.

[21] Mitochondrial fission 1 protein (FIS1) is a mitochondrial outer membrane protein, and as with others (such as mitofusin, VDAC), are targets for Parkin-mediated ubiquitination. By adding ubiquitin molecules to its targets expressed on mitochondria, Parkin normally marks and selects dysfunctional mitochondria for clearance, helping to maintain a functional and healthy mitochondrial network.

## d. Alterations of Intracellular Calcium Homeostasis

Dysregulation of calcium ($Ca^{2+}$) homeostasis has been described in several LSDs; although as with disruption of autophagy, changes have been attributed to various disease-specific mechanisms. Adverse consequences of depleting intracellular $Ca^{2+}$ (in experiments with the cell permeable EGTA-AM) include inhibition of: (1) $H_2O_2$-induced lysosome exocytosis, (2) acid sphingomyelinase (ASM) translocation and (3) the formation of ceramide-enriched platforms [37]. These changes may adversely impact on the process of plasma membrane repair. Interestingly, pharmacological inhibition or genetic deficiency of ASM did not affect $H_2O_2$-induced lysosome exocytosis, which suggests an alternative triggering factor or mechanism.

The aftermath of a disruption in $Ca^{2+}$ homeostasis - *as described below* for several conditions, remains to be clarified by further studies. However, depletion of ER $Ca^{2+}$ is known to cause ER stress and activation of the unfolded protein response machinery, ultimately leading to apoptosis. This process may represent a final common disease pathway for several LSDs.

Elevated intracellular glucosylceramide (GlcCer) levels in Gaucher disease (GD) cellular models has been demonstrated to increase functional $Ca^{2+}$ stores in cultured neurons, which has been related to modulation of ryanodine receptors (an ER $Ca^{2+}$ channel) [38]. Further studies have shown the GlcCer effect was not direct, but achieved through a process possibly involving the redox sensor of the ryanodine receptors (RyaR). The RyaR has also been implicated in $Ca^{2+}$ release resulting from stimulation with galactosylsphingosine (psychosine). Elevated psychosine levels in Krabbe disease has been incriminated in several other deleterious processes (*see* Box 2.7).

A disturbance in intracellular $Ca^{2+}$ also occurs following exposure of cells to the gangliosides $G_{M2}$, $G_{M1}$, and $G_{M3}$. In these instances, elevated cytosolic $Ca^{2+}$ results from the inhibition of uptake via an action on the sarco(endo)plasmic reticulum $Ca^{2+}$-ATPase (SERCA)[22]; observed in neurons and in brain microsomes. Studies have revealed this process requires an

[22] The sarco/endoplasmic reticulum $Ca^{2+}$-ATPase (SERCA) is responsible for transporting $Ca^{2+}$ from the cytosol into the lumen of the sarcoplasmic reticulum following muscular contraction. The $Ca^{2+}$sequestering activity of SERCA facilitates muscular relaxation in both

exposed carboxyl group on the ganglioside sialic acid residue attached to a ceramide backbone [39].

Similarly, dysfunctional acidic $Ca^{2+}$ stores have been observed in Niemann-Pick disease type A (NPD), wherein increased cytosolic $Ca^{2+}$ has been attributed to reduced uptake by SERCA; in this instance, because of low SERCA expression [40]. This is distinct from the observation in $G_{M2}$-gangliosidosis studies, wherein SERCA activity was shown to be inhibited by the excess sialic acid residue of the stored substrate (ganglioside) and not a change in expression levels.

Additionally, in $G_{M1}$-gangliosidosis substrate accumulation in the GSL-enriched fractions of mitochondria-associated ER membranes alters the activity of the $Ca^{2+}$-releasing inositol triphosphate receptor [41]. These changes lead to cytosolic $Ca^{2+}$ overload, and subsequent mitochondrial membrane permeabilization and activation of the mitochondrial apoptosis pathway.

Investigations have revealed alterations of the handling of intracellular $Ca^{2+}$ pools in the endoplasmic reticulum, mitochondria and lysosome in juvenile NCL cells. Administration of thapsigargin led to increased $Ca^{2+}$-mediated SERCA sensitivity and autophagosome accumulation in affected cells, which could be reversed by $Ca^{2+}$ chelation [42]. These findings support an important role for the cognate (CLN3) protein in intracellular $Ca^{2+}$ handling and in autophagic pathway flux.

In Niemann-Pick disease type C1 (NPC1), lysosomal accumulation of sphingosine leads to a decrease in lysosomal $Ca^{2+}$ and reduced NAADP-mediated $Ca^{2+}$ release; which has a negative effect on endosomal-lysosome fusion and trafficking within the cell. As a consequence, there is secondary accumulation of cholesterol, sphingomyelin, and glycosphingolipids. Thapsigargin (a SERCA pump inhibitor) and curcumin have been shown to improve trafficking and reduce pathology in NPC1 cells; in the mouse model of NPC1, treatment with curcumin (which induces endogenous antioxidant defense mechanisms and exhibits anti-inflammatory activity) slowed the rate of disease progression and increased survival [43].

The cellular mechanisms underlying disruption of $Ca^{2+}$ homeostasis may vary among the LSDs, but restoration of cytosolic and organelle $Ca^{2+}$ to physiologic levels may be a potential adjunctive therapeutic approach.

---

cardiac and skeletal muscle. Impaired function of SERCA has emerged as a major contributor to ER stress.

A recent report describes the lysosomal expression of big-conductance $Ca^{2+}$-activated potassium (BK) channels that physically and functionally couple with TRPML1,[23] a lysosomal $Ca^{2+}$ release channel; defects of which cause mucolipidosis type IV. BK overexpression was shown to rescue the secondary impairment of TRPML1-mediated $Ca^{2+}$ release and abnormal lysosomal storage in NPC1 cells [44].

## e. Cell Death, Inappropriate Apoptosis and Necroptosis

Cell death in response to various insults can be categorized as apoptotic or necrotic, which when excessive or uncontrolled can trigger an innate immune response; a vicious cycle resulting in further loss of cells. These cell death pathways are characterized by associated morphological changes and core molecules that have a regulatory role and function as 'effectors'.

Apoptosis engages the caspase family of intracellular cysteine proteases, promoting the dismantling of the cell into membrane-enveloped fragments ('apoptotic bodies') that are then rapidly cleared by surrounding healthy cells [45]. CED-9 and EGL-1 are members of the BCL-2 family of pro-apoptotic proteins which are the principal regulators of the intrinsic apoptotic pathway (involving the permeabilization of the outer mitochondrial membrane). In contrast, the extrinsic pathway is triggered when cell-surface death receptors (such as Fas) are bound by their ligands. Both pathways draw in the caspase family of 'effectors'.

Progressive apoptotic loss of photoreceptor cells has been observed in the neuronal ceroid lipofuscinosis CLN6 mouse model. Specifically, a reduction of the outer nuclear layer (to approximately 3 rows of photoreceptor cells) was found at 9 months of age [46], although signs of reactive gliosis were observed earlier (i.e., in 1-month-old affected mice). Ultrastructural analysis revealed lysosomal storage material containing curvilinear and fingerprint-like inclusions in various retinal cell types. Examination of retinal cells from affected mice revealed increased expression levels of soluble mannose 6-

[23] Normally, $Ca^{2+}$ from lysosomes is released via TRPML1 through activation of BK channels, which in turn facilitates further lysosomal $Ca^{2+}$ release and membrane trafficking. The mammalian target of rapamycin (mTOR), a nutrient-sensitive protein kinase that negatively

phosphate-containing lysosomal enzymes (such as cathepsin D) and the lysosomal membrane protein LAMP1.

Programmed necrosis ('necroptosis') is initiated by cell death receptors (such as the pro-inflammatory tumor necrosis factor receptor 1 (TNFR1), which requires the serine-threonine kinase activity of receptor-interacting protein 1 (RIP1; also known as RIPK1) and RIP3 (RIPK3) [47]. Its implementation takes place independent of the pro-apoptotic caspase-8, and involves the active disintegration of organelle (i.e., mitochondria and lysosome) and plasma membranes. Necroptosis as a mechanism of cell death has been described in two of the glycosphingolipidoses: Gaucher disease and Krabbe disease [48].

So-called lysosomal cell death is triggered by lysosomal membrane permeabilization (LMP) and the subsequent release of lysosomal hydrolases from the lysosomal lumen into the cytosol. In the cytosol, lysosomal cathepsin proteases act as executioners for cell death-either autonomously without caspase activation or in concert with the classical apoptotic machinery [49].

Endogenous agents that can cause LMP include reactive oxygen species (ROS) and lipid metabolites such as sphingosine and phosphatidic acid. Conversely, lysosomal sphingomyelin and cholesterol accumulation characteristic of Niemann-Pick disease impairs LMP. In this instance, cellular dysfunction may be due to other factors; but as LMP (within bounds) can be part of normal homeostatic events, its impairment may also eventually be damaging to the cell.

## f. Metabolic and Oxidative Stress Response

Metabolic stress responses (also referred to as heat shock response, HSR) can be induced in reaction to a number of physiological and pathological stresses, such as protein misfolding and aggregation, endoplasmic reticulum stress (with changes in intracellular $Ca^{2+}$ concentration) and oxidative stress (with mitochondrial dysregulation). The cytoprotective actions of the HSR include processes involving the lysosomal system, such as cell death and autophagy, as a means of clearing non-salvageable defective cells; and protection against lysosomal membrane permeabilization, in potentially viable

regulates autophagy, directly targets and inactivates the TRPML1 channel and thereby functional autophagy.

cells [51]. As with other homeostatic mechanisms when unregulated, HSR can be detrimental and lead to cell death; ultimately via apoptosis.

Oxidative stress represents a lack of balance between reactive oxygen/nitrogen species production and the anti-oxidant system. Brain tissue is particularly vulnerable to oxidative stress for several reasons: (1) high $O_2$ consumption, (2) high tissue concentration of iron (leading to production of reactive oxygen species, in the so-called Fenton reaction), (3) presence of excitatory amino acids and dopamine metabolism (which generate hydrogen peroxide), and (4) low levels of antioxidant defenses [52]. Polyunsaturated fatty acids (PUFA), such as linoleic acid and arachidonic acid, are abundant lipids within neuronal membranes; representing principal targets of oxidation (attributed to the presence of one or several nucleophilic unsaturated double bonds) [53].

Studies in the infantile NCL (*PPT1*-knockout) mice have described neuronal death by apoptosis, which is in part caused by endoplasmic reticulum (ER) and oxidative stresses. Affected fibroblasts from patients with distinct NCL showed increased sensitivity to brefeldin-A-induced apoptosis, which suggested pre-existing ER stress levels [54]. Quantitation of mRNA levels of both ER (i.e., ATF6, calnexin, Grp78, and XBP1) *and* oxidative stress (i.e., superoxide dismutase-2, catalase, and thiotransferase-1) markers revealed consistently higher values, compared with control. In these studies, administration of chemical chaperones alleviated ER and oxidative stresses, and was as noted to be cytoprotective.

To ascertain links between oxidative stress and inflammation, analysis of relevant markers in the brain cortex of MPS-IIIB mice was undertaken, and results compared with findings in unaffected control mice and double mutant TLR4 knockout (KO)-MPS-IIIB mice. [TLR4 was chosen for its determinant role in early-onset inflammation present in MPS-IIIB cortex]. Oxidative stress was evident at a very early stage in the brain of affected mice [26]. These observations were deemed not to be a consequence of neuroinflammation but an independent phenomenon, as the enzymatic activity of total superoxide dismutase (SOD) was already greater in the cortex of 10-day-old double mutant MPS-IIIB/TLR4-null mice, when there were no detectable signs of inflammation. At 3 and 8 months of age, the total enzymatic activities of glutathione peroxidase, SOD, and carbonyl protein levels in the cortex of affected double-KO mice were similar to those measured in mice with MPS-IIIB alone at a stage when signs of inflammation was present; in both disease-mice models, associated changes were higher than those observed in controls.

These observations indicated no added impact attributable to inflammatory processes over time. Thus, the reactive oxygen species production (in direct response to heparan sulfate accumulation), which leads to oxidative damage and protein oxidation in particular, appears to be primary and an early event in the causation of cellular dysfunction during neurodegeneration in the MPS-IIIB mouse model.

It is likely the different pathologies discussed in this chapter represent interlocking phenomena leading to cell death; although it can be anticipated particular events occur in a cell-type specific manner and in a temporal fashion (i.e., related to developmental stage). Currently, it is not certain which of these factors play a dominant role; nor the sequence of their occurrence, in cases wherein there are two or more findings. Ultimately, metabolomic studies and analysis of metabolite flux may shed more light on these phenomena. What is evident is the central role of the lysosome, as a hub for several homeostatic mechanisms; and that a disruption of these processes leads ultimately to disease, triggered in the case of LSDs by progressive storage of incompletely metabolized substrates that serve a persistent activator. A summary of disease mechanisms implicated in the LSDs is shown in Table 2.2.

**Table 2.2. Disease mechanisms implicated in various LSDs**

| Disease | Inflammation | Autophagy dysfunction | Altered $Ca^{2+}$ homeostasis | Lysolipid accumulation |
|---|---|---|---|---|
| Mucopolysaccharidosis: | | | | |
| I | + | | | |
| III | + | + | | |
| VI | + | | | |
| VII | + | | | |
| Multiple sulphatase deficiency | + | + | | |
| Sphingolipidosis: | | | | |
| Fabry | | | | + |
| Gaucher | + | | + | + |
| $G_{M1}$-gangliosidosis | + | + | + | + |
| $G_{M2}$-gangliosidosis | + | | + | + |
| Krabbe | + | | | + |
| Niemann-Pick A | | | + | |
| Niemann-Pick C | + | + | | |
| Glycogenosis: | | | | |
| Pompe | | + | | |

**Box 2.1. Phenotype variability and putative modifying factors**

Genotype-phenotype studies have been undertaken in several LSDs, but most of these have revealed a lack of perfect concordance, which indicates a role for modifying factors; although in most instances these have not been defined.

In Gaucher disease (GD), *GBA* mutation analyses has revealed two common disease alleles across various populations (i.e., c.1226A > G, p.Asn409Ser, N370S) and c.1448T > C, p.Leu483Pro, L444P), except among Asians in whom the c.1226A > G allele is rare; this latter fact may account for the greater proportion of patients with neuropathic features in these communities.

Patients with at least one c.1226A > G allele do not develop the neurodegenerative features associated with severe GD types II and III, although it does not eliminate the risk for Parkinson disease. Patients with the c.1448T > C allele tend to have severe disease, marked by neuropathic features when associated with another deleterious mutation other than c.1226A > G. Patients with GD homozygous for the c.1342G > C (p.Asp448His, D409H) mutation, first described among the Jenin-Arab population, have a unique life-limiting cardiovascular complication: aortic and mitral valve calcification, which tends to develop during the peripubertal period. In the Balkan region, this mutation is found in *cis* (i.e., on the same allele) with the c.882T > G mutation (p.His294Gln, H255Q); in these cases (i.e., homozygotes for c.1342G > C/c.882T > G mutations) the condition manifests as severe GD type II. Therapy with HSCT and ERT has not been shown to alter ultimate neurologic prognosis, and thus is not indicated for GD type II; ERT in GD type III (which can be associated with survival into 30's and beyond) can have a significant positive impact on quality of life for affected individuals.

Recent studies have shown *CLN8* expression may influence GD severity: with increased expression of the *CLN8* gene potentially protective against severe GD type I manifestations. In cultured skin fibroblasts from affected patients homozygous for the c.1226A > G mutation, the relative expression of *CLN8* was higher in mild GD patients compared to severe cases; in whom certain *CLN8* risk alleles were overrepresented. The mechanistic basis of these observations is not known, but potentially the *CLN8* gene product may function as a protective sphingolipid sensor and/or have a positive influence glycosphingolipid trafficking.

The *CLN8* gene encodes an ER protein that shares domain homology with ceramide (Cer) synthases. Mutations in the *CLN8* gene which lead to loss of function is the cause of late-infantile neuronal ceroid lipofuscinosis. Interestingly, studies have revealed reduced Cer and Galactosyl-Cer levels in the brain of these patients and affected mice.

**Suggested readings:**

*Grabowski GA, Zimran A, Ida H. 2015. Gaucher disease types 1 and 3: Phenotypic characterization of large populations from the ICGG Gaucher Registry. Am J Hematol. 90 Suppl 1:S12-8.*

*Santamaria R, Michelakakis H, Moraitou M, Dimitriou E, Dominissini S, Grossi S, Sánchez-Ollé G, Chabás A, Pittis MG, Filocamo M, Vilageliu L, Grinberg D. 2008. Haplotype analysis suggests a single Balkan origin for the Gaucher disease [D409H;H255Q] double mutant allele. Hum Mutat. 29(6):E58-67.*

*Zhang CK, Stein PB, Liu J, Wang Z, Yang R, Cho JH, Gregersen PK, Aerts JM, Zhao H, Pastores GM, Mistry PK. 2012. Genome-wide association study of N370S homozygous Gaucher disease reveals the candidacy of CLN8 gene as a genetic modifier contributing to extreme phenotypic variation. Am J Hematol. 87(4):377-83.*

**Box 2.2. Activators/Co-factors involved with glycosphingolipid metabolism** *(see Figure 2.2)*

The catabolism of glycosphingolipids with short oligosaccharide chains requires the presence of membrane-active lysosomal lipid-binding proteins; known as saposins.

- Saposin A: physiological activator of β-galactosylceramidase. Accordingly, mutations result in symptoms that are similar to Krabbe disease.
- Saposin B: activator of sulfatide; underlying defects is the cause of a rare metachromatic leukodystrophy (MLD) variant in which arylsulfatase A (ARSA) activity is normal.
- Prosaposin (*PSAP*) gene which affects Saposin C (which normally promotes the accessibility of the GlcCer substrate to β-glucosidase: can lead to a visceral, non-neuronopathic or type III-like Gaucher disease.
- Saposin D: normally serves as an activator of acid ceramidase; a deficiency of saposin D in mice results in Cer storage and cerebellar Purkinje cell degeneration.

The saposins are situated at the surface of intraluminal lysosomal vesicles, facilitating the interaction between the relevant hydrolases and its sphingolipid substrate (embedded in the membrane of inner endolysosomal vesicles). This process is strongly stimulated by membrane lipids, enriched in anionic bis(monoacylglycero)phosphate (BMP). The individual sphingolipid activator proteins or saposins (A-D) are encoded by the prosaposin (*PSAP*) gene. Investigations of prosaposin trafficking to lysosomes led to discovery of the lysosomal sorting receptor, sortilin. Prosaposin is also secreted to the extracellular space as oligomers, wherein it exerts a variety of nervous tissues responses including the activation of G protein-coupled receptors and ERK phosphorylation.

**Suggested readings:**

*Carvelli L, Libin Y, Morales CR.2015. Prosaposin: a protein with differential sorting and multiple functions. Histol Histopathol. 30(6):647-60.*
*Schulze H, Sandhoff K. 2014. Sphingolipids and lysosomal pathologies. Biochim Biophys Acta. 1841(5):799-810.*

**Box 2.3. Substrate biosynthetic defects**

*(see Figure 2.3)*

Substrate synthesis inhibition is a potential therapeutic approach for certain LSDs *(discussed in the next chapter)*. Insights into the normal roles of certain molecules which end up as substrates in the lysosome (for clearance or recycling) have been obtained from studies of genes whose protein products are involved with the biosynthesis of glycosphingolipids (GSL, composed of an oligosaccharide headgroup linked to a ceramide backbone). GSLs are mainly synthesized in the Golgi and transported to other destinations within the cell. These biosynthetic defects are separate conditions and are not classified as LSDs.

$G_{M3}$ synthase (encoded by *ST3GAL5*) is the first biosynthetic enzyme of a- and b-series gangliosides. Loss-of-function *ST3GAL5* mutations have been shown to cause autosomal recessive (AR) infantile-onset epilepsy associated with developmental stagnation. Associated features include occipital white matter abnormalities, cortical atrophy and abnormally pigmented skin.

*ST3GAL5* mutations leading to an unstable $G_{M3}$ synthase have been associated with a different clinical picture: the so-called 'salt-and-pepper' syndrome with altered dermal pigmentation; associated features include facial dysmorphism, seizures, severe intellectual disability, spasticity, and choreoathetosis. The corresponding mouse model displays behavioural changes and hearing loss. It is hypothesized $G_{M3}$-dependent membrane microdomains might be essential for the proper organization and maintenance of stereocilia in auditory hair cells.

*B4GALNT1* encodes the enzyme $G_{M2}$ synthase which catalyses the second step in complex ganglioside biosynthesis. *B4GALNT1* mutations cause an AR form of spastic paraplegia (SPG26), characterized by progressive weakness and spasticity affecting the lower and, in some cases, the upper extremities. Patients may also present with moderate cognitive impairment, cerebellar signs, sensory neuropathy, and psychiatric symptoms. Brain MRI may reveal cortical or subcortical atrophy.

*FA2H* encodes an enzyme that introduces a hydroxyl group at the C2-position of fatty acids, which are subsequently incorporated by ceramide synthases into sphingolipids and galactolipids (the substrate which accumulates in Krabbe disease). 2-hydroxylation of sphingolipids is deemed to help with stabilizing the lateral interactions of membranes. Mutations of *FA2H* are associated with a progressive AR disorder characterized by white matter degeneration consistent with spastic paraplegia (SPG35), leukodystrophy or neurodegeneration associated with brain iron accumulation (NBIA).

**Suggested readings:**

*Boccuto L, Aoki K, Flanagan-Steet H, Chen CF, Fan X, Bartel F, Petukh M, Pittman A, Saul R, Chaubey A, Alexov E, Tiemeyer M, Steet R, Schwartz CE. 2014. A mutation in a ganglioside biosynthetic enzyme, ST3GAL5, results in salt and pepper syndrome, a neurocutaneous disorder with altered glycolipid and glycoprotein glycosylation. Hum Mol Genet. 23(2):418-33.*

*Harlalka GV, Lehman A, Chioza B, Baple EL, Maroofian R, Cross H, Sreekantan-Nair A, Priestman DA, Al-Turki S, McEntagart ME, Proukakis C, Royle L, Kozak RP, Bastaki L, Patton M, Wagner K, Coblentz R, Price J, Mezei M, Schlade-Bartusiak K, Platt FM, Hurles ME, Crosby AH. 2013. Mutations in B4GALNT1 (GM2 synthase) underlie a new disorder of ganglioside biosynthesis. Brain. 136(Pt 12):3618-24.*

*Wakil SM, Monies DM, Ramzan K, Hagos S, Bastaki L, Meyer BF, Bohlega S. 2014. Novel B4GALNT1 mutations in a complicated form of hereditary spastic paraplegia. Clin Genet.86(5):500-1.*

*Yoshikawa M, Go S, Suzuki S, Katori Y, Morlet T, Gottlieb SM, Fujiwara M, Iwasaki K, Strauss KA, Inokuchi J. 2015. Ganglioside GM3 is essential for the structural integrity and function of cochlear hair cells. Hum Mol Genet. 24(10):2796-807.*

**Box 2.4. Biomarkers and Lysosomal storage diseases**

A biological marker (or biomarker) is a substance (analyte) in tissue or fluids (e.g., chitotriosidase), or alternatively a clinical sign (e.g., myocardial fibrosis) that is an objective indication of a medical state.

Characteristics of an ideal biomarker:

- Significant elevation (in concentration or activity) with disease, and no overlap in values between untreated patients and healthy subjects. In this instance, the biomarker may be potentially useful in screening target populations to identify undiagnosed cases (e.g., elevated oxysterols in screening for NPC cases).
- Correlation with total body burden of disease, or specific organ involvement,
  - With its concentration or activity changing in relation to disease progression, or
  - Changes that occur in response to treatment; best when it parallels key clinical endpoints (i.e., useful as a surrogate)
- Moreover, concentration or activity should not vary in response to factors unrelated to disease or non-specific therapy (i.e., not aimed at underlying biochemical defect); and
- Can be objectively measured - quickly, reliably, and cheaply; in easily accessible body fluids, such as blood, CSF or urine.

Marked heterogeneity in clinical expression and disease course can be a challenge when providing genetic counselling to newly diagnosed patients and their relatives, and also when offering a prognosis and treatment recommendations, if indicated. Thus, informative biomarkers may help refine counselling, to complement knowledge of patient's genotype.

Chitotriosidase (a chitinase) was found to be elevated in patients with Gaucher disease (GD); secreted by Gaucher cells (i.e., lipid-engorged macrophage). Studies have shown plasma chitotriosidase (CHIT1) activity provides a rough estimate of body burden of Gaucher cells.

Reductions in plasma chitotriosidase during therapy have been shown to correlate significantly with reductions in liver and spleen volumes; trends have also been noted with improvements in haemoglobin and platelet count, and the reconstitution of bone marrow composition.

Among patients with GD, the occurrence of long-term complications and associated conditions such as multiple myeloma, osteonecrosis, Parkinson disease, hepatocellular carcinoma and pulmonary hypertension have been positively correlated with (1) baseline plasma chitotriosidase levels (i.e., pre-enzyme therapy); (2) the average plasma chitotriosidase level during 3 years of ERT; and (3) residual plasma chitotriosidase after 2 years of ERT.

Approximately 6% and 35% of individuals are homozygous or heterozygous, respectively, for the most common polymorphism in the CHIT1 gene, a 24-bp duplication (dup-24 bp). Homozygosity for the dup-24 bp allele leads to inactivation of chitotriosidase enzyme activity but without major consequences for health. [The latter indicates, it is not a factor which exerts an influence on GD phenotype.] In patients null for CHIT1, the marker PARK/CCL18 has been measured, and shown to parallel clinical observations made with observed chitotriosidase values.

**Suggested readings:**

*Deegan PB, Moran MT, McFarlane I, Schofield JP, Boot RG, Aerts JM, Cox TM. 2005. Clinical evaluation of chemokine and enzymatic biomarkers of Gaucher disease. Blood Cells Mol Dis. 35(2):259-67.*

*van Dussen L, Hendriks EJ, Groener JE, Boot RG, Hollak CE, Aerts JM. 2014. Value of plasma chitotriosidase to assess non-neuronopathic Gaucher disease severity and progression in the era of enzyme replacement therapy. J Inherit Metab Dis. 37(6):991-1001.*

## Box 2.5. Lipid rafts: Glycosphingolipid topology and organization

Glycosphinglolipids (GSL) have tightly packed backbones, and exhibit preferential interaction with each other and with sphingomyelin and cholesterol in a phospholipid environment to form *lipid rafts*. Glycosylated molecules on the cell surface are involved in the formation of 'glycosynapse', formed by two opposed lipid rafts, where binding selectively depends on GSL-GSL interactions. These interfaces have roles in myelin formation, maintenance and function. Additionally, ceramides, generated from sphingomyelin metabolism, are implicated in the formation of ceramide-enriched microdomains and membrane remodelling events.

Galactosylceramide and sulfatide on opposing surfaces of myelin sheaths interact with each other, enabling the compaction and formation of mature myelin. Myelin, which encloses segments of axons, is formed by oligodendrocytes and Schwann cells in the central and peripheral nervous system, respectively.

These dynamic lipid domains in plasma membranes recruit proteins and other lipids, and serve as an organizing platform. Lipid domains influence membrane fluidity and are involved with regulating transmembrane signalling. Studies have shown $G_{M1}$-gangliosides are enriched in caveolae (specialized-lipid rafts enriched in GSLs and integral membrane proteins known as caveolin, which are stabilized by a protein scaffold comprised of cavins). Interactions within these discrete domains involve modulation of cell-type specific ion transport, neuronal differentiation, G protein-coupled receptor activation, immune system reactivity and neuroprotective signalling.

Various biological ligands (e.g., toxins, lectins, viruses or bacteria) bind to glycolipids on the cell surface and induce their uptake into cells by creating membrane invaginations. Several pathogens hijack plasma membrane receptors, often associated with lipid rafts, to gain entry into cells and create havoc. Globotriaosylceramide (the lipid which accumulates in Fabry disease) is implicated in the action of the Shiga toxin. Recently, it has been shown that newly synthesized hepatitis A virus (HAV) particles accumulate in lysosomal organelles and that lysosomal enzymes are involved in the maturation cleavage of the virion. Inhibiting the processes of fusion of lysosomes with the plasma membrane promoted the nonlytic release of HAV from infected cells.

**Suggested readings:**

*Aigal S, Claudinon J, Römer W. 2015. Plasma membrane reorganization: A glycolipid gateway for microbes. Biochim Biophys Acta. 1853(4):858-71.*

*Aureli M, Grassi S, Prioni S, Sonnino S, Prinetti A. 2015. Lipid membrane domains in the brain. Biochim Biophys Acta. 1851(8):1006-16.*

*Ledeen RW, Wu G. 2015. The multi-tasked life of $G_{M1}$ ganglioside, a true factotum of nature. Trends Biochem Sci. 40(7):407-418.*

*Seggewiß N, Paulmann D, Dotzauer A. 2014. Lysosomes serve as a platform for hepatitis A virus particle maturation and nonlytic release. Arch Virol. PMID: 26467925.*

*van Meer G, Hoetzl S. 2010. Sphingolipid topology and the dynamic organization and function of membrane proteins. FEBS Lett. 584(9):1800-5.*

## Box 2.6. Autophagy-Lysosomal Pathways implicated in

Parkinson disease (PD), an age-related neurodegenerative condition, is associated with the accumulation of α-synuclein (SNCA) and loss of dopaminergic neurons in the substantia nigra pars compacta. SNCA is an autophagy substrate (mediated by interactions with LAMP2A and the chaperone HSPA8); defective SNCA clearance by various mechanisms may be a convergent point ultimately leading up to the disease.

Initially thought to be mainly a sporadic disorder, several gene defects have been identified as risk or causal factors. At least 11 of the implicated genes are integral to autophagy-lysosomal processes: *LRRK2, GBA, SMPD1, SCARB2 (LIMP2), SNCA, PARK2, PINK1, PARK7, LAMP3, RAB29/RAB7L1, MAPT, GAK, SREBF1, GPNMB,* and potentially *TMEM175.* Across a diverse population of individuals, *LRRK2* (1-5%) and *GBA* (3-20%) gene defects represent the two most common risk factors for PD, although both loci are associated with reduced penetrance (i.e., the proportion of carriers developing clinical manifestations). Altogether, these observations suggest a critical role of lysosomal dysfunction in the development of neurodegenerative disorders, likely operative in concert with other deleterious events that occur in senescent cells.

***GBA*** encodes the lysosomal enzyme β-glucosidase (GC); bi-allelic gene defects lead to Gaucher disease. Individuals with one (carrier) or two *GBA* mutations have an increased risk of developing PD. Reduced enzyme activity is believed to promote SNCA aggregation (the major constituent of **Lewy bodies**), which in turn further inhibits GC activity (in a deleterious feedback loop). Severe *GBA* mutations tend to be associated with an earlier age of PD onset.

***SCARB2 (LIMP2)*** encodes the scavenger receptor class B, member 2 protein, responsible for targeting of nascent GC to the lysosome; recessive defects are the cause progressive myoclonic epilepsy and renal failure.

***SMPD1*** encodes the lysosomal enzyme acid sphingomyelinase; bi-allelic gene defects lead to Niemann-Pick (type A/B) disease. Individuals with one (carrier) *SMPD1* mutation have an increased risk of developing PD. Reduced enzyme activity results in a disruption of ceramide metabolism, which has implications for the regulation of autophagy.

***LRRK2*** encodes leucine-rich repeat kinase 2; defects of the cognate protein impair its interaction with LAMP2A (a CMA receptor) and disrupts chaperone-mediated autophagy (CMA). Increased GTPase activity of LRRK2 has been shown to impair endocytic vesicular trafficking and autophagy.

***PINK1*** and ***PARK2*** encode proteins involved with selective mitochondrial engulfment by autophagosomes and their degradation within lysosomes, which is facilitated by CTSD.

**Suggested reading**

*Gan-Or Z, Dion PA, Rouleau GA. 2015. Genetic perspective on the role of the Autophagy-Lysosome Pathway in Parkinson disease. Autophagy. Jul 24:0.*

**Box 2.7. Psychosine-mediated toxicity**

Galactosylsphingosine (psychosine) is a constituent of cerebrosides, normally formed from UDP-galactose and sphingosine by UDP-galactose-sphingosine β-D-galactosyltransferase. It is unusual in being a basic (cationic) lipid with a detergent-like structure, so it has binding properties that differ from those of other lipids.

Psychosine has been found to be elevated in Krabbe disease (KD); likely due to deacylation of galactosylceramide (the primary substrate which builds up in this condition). Several studies have described the deleterious consequences of elevated psychosine, such as: (1) cell death associated with induction of pro-inflammatory cytokines (e.g., tumor necrosis factor-α and interleukin-6); (2) induction of nitric oxide synthase activity, and lysophosphatidylcholine generation; (3) down-regulation of the phosphoinositide 3-kinase (PI3K)-Akt survival pathway; (4) expression of prostaglandin D synthase; and (5) formation of multinuclear globoid-like cells in U937 monocytic cells (which has been attributed to inhibition of cytokinesis, and not by cell–cell fusion).

Psychosine-induced cell death of oligodendrocytes may involve the phospholipase A2 (PLA2)-mediated signal transduction pathway. Apoptotic cells and expression of apoptosis-related molecules such as TNF-α and its receptor-1 have been observed in *twitcher* mice and brains of patients with KD, providing confirmation *in vivo* of some of the changes largely cell-based studies described in the preceding paragraph. Increased connexin 43 has also been implicated in cell death of oligodendrocyte precursors induced by psychosine.

The relationship between apoptosis and psychosine-mediated stress signal also can be explained by MAPKs that act by down-regulating the prosurvival (NF-κB) and up-regulating the stress-mediated signal transduction pathways (JNK/AP-1) with or without the receptor function.

Moreover, psychosine has been found to (1) down-regulate AMP-activated protein kinase (AMPK), which leads to induction of inflammation in astrocytes without directly affecting oligodendrocyte cell death; and (2) inhibit the activity of protein kinase C. Psychosine has also been identified as an endothelial actin-disassembling agent endowed with anti-angiogenic activity *in vitro* and *in vivo*.

Added psychosine-mediated toxic effects point to mitochondria dysfunction, including inhibition of the electron transport chain, loss of mitochondrial membrane potential, alteration of oxidative phosphorylation, cytochrome c release and activation of caspases 3 and 9.

These observations point to multiple pathways leading to cellular dysfunction, or loss (necroptosis). It is likely some changes will turn out to be cell-type specific. Further studies may provide insights into ways of neutralizing these detrimental effects.

**Suggested readings:**

*Claycomb KI, Winokur PN, Johnson KM, Nicaise AM, Giampetruzzi AW, Sacino AV, Snyder EY, Barbarese E, Bongarzone ER, Crocker SJ. 2014.. Aberrant production of tenascin-C in globoid cell leukodystrophy alters psychosine-induced microglial functions. J Neuropathol Exp Neurol. 73(10):964-74.*

*Graziano AC, Parenti R, Avola R, Cardile V. 2015. Krabbe disease: involvement of connexin43 in the apoptotic effects of sphingolipid psychosine on mouse oligodendrocyte precursors. Apoptosis. PMID: 26459425*

*O'Sullivan C, Dev KK. 2015. Galactosylsphingosine (psychosine)-induced demyelination is attenuated by sphingosine 1-phosphate signalling. J Cell Sci. 128(21):3878-87.*

*Voccoli V, Tonazzini I, Signore G, Caleo M, Cecchini M. 2014. Role of extracellular calcium and mitochondrial oxygen species in psychosine-induced oligodendrocyte cell death. Cell Death Dis. 5:e1529.*

# References

[1] Clarke LA. 2011. Pathogenesis of skeletal and connective tissue involvement in the mucopolysaccharidoses: glycosaminoglycan storage is merely the instigator. *Rheumatology* (Oxford). 50 Suppl 5:v13-8.

[2] Novinec M, Lenarčič B, Turk B. 2014. Cysteine cathepsin activity regulation by glycosaminoglycans. *Biomed Res Int*. 2014:309718.

[3] Salazar DA, Rodríguez-López A, Herreño A, Barbosa H, Herrera J, Ardila A, Barreto GE, González J, Alméciga-Díaz CJ. 2015. Systems biology study of mucopolysaccharidosis using a human metabolic reconstruction network. *Mol Genet Metab*. S1096-7192(15)30036-6.

[4] Zhou K, Blom T. 2015. Trafficking and Functions of Bioactive Sphingolipids: Lessons from Cells and Model Membranes. *Lipid Insights*. 8(Suppl 1):11-20.

[5] McGlynn R, Dobrenis K, Walkley SU. 2004. Differential subcellular localization of cholesterol, gangliosides, and glycosaminoglycans in

murine models of mucopolysaccharide storage disorders. *J Comp Neurol.* 480(4):415-26.

[6] Lamanna WC, Lawrence R, Sarrazin S, Esko JD. 2011. Secondary storage of dermatan sulfate in Sanfilippo disease. *J Biol Chem.* 286(9):6955-62.

[7] Woloszynek JC, Coleman T, Semenkovich CF, Sands MS. 2007. Lysosomal dysfunction results in altered energy balance. *J Biol Chem.* 282(49):35765-71.

[8] Woloszynek JC, Kovacs A, Ohlemiller KK, Roberts M, Sands MS. 2009. Metabolic adaptations to interrupted glycosaminoglycan recycling. *J Biol Chem.* 284(43):29684-91.

[9] Kooper AJ, Janssens PM, de Groot AN, Liebrand-van Sambeek ML, van den Berg CJ, Tan-Sindhunata GB, van den Berg PP, Bijlsma EK, Smits AP, Wevers RA. 2006. Lysosomal storage diseases in non-immune hydrops fetalis pregnancies. *Clin Chim Acta.* 371(1-2):176-82.

[10] Walkley SU. 2003. Neurobiology and cellular pathogenesis of glycolipid storage diseases. *Philos Trans R Soc Lond B Biol Sci.* 358(1433):893-904.

[11] Passafaro M, Nakagawa T, Sala C, Sheng M. 2003. Induction of dendritic spines by an extracellular domain of AMPA receptor subunit GluR2. *Nature.* 424(6949):677-81.

[12] Saglietti L, Dequidt C, Kamieniarz K, Rousset MC, Valnegri P, Thoumine O, Beretta F, Fagni L, Choquet D, Sala C, Sheng M, Passafaro M. 2007. Extracellular interactions between GluR2 and N-cadherin in spine regulation. *Neuron.* 54(3):461-77.

[13] Zhu Y, Matsumoto T, Nagasawa T, Mackay F, Murakami F. 2015. Chemokine Signalling Controls Integrity of Radial Glial Scaffold in Developing Spinal Cord and Consequential Proper Position of Boundary Cap Cells. *J Neurosci.* 35(24):9211-24.

[14] Uchihara T, Ohashi K, Kitagawa M, Kurata M, Nakamura A, Hirokawa K, Kasuga T, Kobayashi T. 2010. Sialidosis type I carrying V217M/G243R mutations in lysosomal sialidase: an autopsy study demonstrating terminal sialic acid in lysosomal lamellar inclusions and cerebellar dysplasia. *Acta Neuropathol.* 119(1):135-45.

[15] Annunziata I, Patterson A, Helton D, Hu H, Moshiach S, Gomero E, Nixon R, d'Azzo A. 2013. Lysosomal NEU1 deficiency affects amyloid precursor protein levels and amyloid-β secretion via deregulated lysosomal exocytosis. *Nat Commun.* 4:2734.

[16] Kielar C, Wishart TM, Palmer A, Dihanich S, Wong AM, Macauley SL, Chan CH, Sands MS, Pearce DA, Cooper JD, Gillingwater TH. 2009. Molecular correlates of axonal and synaptic pathology in mouse models of Batten disease. *Hum Mol Genet*. 18(21):4066-80.

[17] Wilkinson FL, Holley RJ, Langford-Smith KJ, Badrinath S, Liao A, Langford-Smith A, Cooper JD, Jones SA, Wraith JE, Wynn RF, Merry CL, Bigger BW. 2012. Neuropathology in mouse models of mucopolysaccharidosis type I, IIIA and IIIB. *PLoS One*. 7(4):e35787.

[18] Vitry S, Ausseil J, Hocquemiller M, Bigou S, Dos Santos Coura R, Heard JM. 2009. Enhanced degradation of synaptophysin by the proteasome in mucopolysaccharidosis type IIIB. *Mol Cell Neurosci*. 41(1):8-18.

[19] Bruyère J, Roy E, Ausseil J, Lemonnier T, Teyre G, Bohl D, Etienne-Manneville S, Lortat-Jacob H, Heard JM, Vitry S. 2015. Heparan sulfate saccharides modify focal adhesions: implication in mucopoly-saccharidosis neuropathophysiology. *J Mol Biol*. 427(4):775-91.

[20] Ohmi K, Zhao HZ, Neufeld EF. 2011. Defects in the medial entorhinal cortex and dentate gyrus in the mouse model of Sanfilippo syndrome type B. *PLoS One*. 6(11):e27461.

[21] Lojewski X, Staropoli JF, Biswas-Legrand S, Simas AM, Haliw L, Selig MK, Coppel SH, Goss KA, Petcherski A, Chandrachud U, Sheridan SD, Lucente D, Sims KB, Gusella JF, Sondhi D, Crystal RG, Reinhardt P, Sterneckert J, Schöler H, Haggarty SJ, Storch A, Hermann A, Cotman SL. 2014. Human iPSC models of neuronal ceroid lipofuscinosis capture distinct effects of TPP1 and CLN3 mutations on the endocytic pathway. *Hum Mol Genet*. 23(8):2005-22.

[22] Plati T, Visigalli I, Capotondo A, Buono M, Naldini L, Cosma MP, Biffi A. 2009. Development and maturation of invariant NKT cells in the presence of lysosomal engulfment. *Eur J Immunol*. 39(10):2748-54.

[23] Gadola SD, Silk JD, Jeans A, Illarionov PA, Salio M, Besra GS, Dwek R, Butters TD, Platt FM, Cerundolo V. 2006. Impaired selection of invariant natural killer T cells in diverse mouse models of glycosphingolipid lysosomal storage diseases. *J Exp Med*. 203(10):2293-303.

[24] Cartier N, Lewis CA, Zhang R, Rossi FM. 2014. The role of microglia in human disease: therapeutic tool or target? *Acta Neuropathol*. 128(3):363-80.

[25] Ausseil J, Desmaris N, Bigou S, Attali R, Corbineau S, Vitry S, Parent M, Cheillan D, Fuller M, Maire I, Vanier MT, Heard JM. 2008. Early neurodegeneration progresses independently of microglial activation by heparan sulfate in the brain of mucopolysaccharidosis IIIB mice. *PLoS One*. 3(5):e2296.

[26] Trudel S, Trécherel E, Gomila C, Peltier M, Aubignat M, Gubler B, Morlière P, Heard JM, Ausseil J. 2015. Oxidative stress is independent of inflammation in the neurodegenerative Sanfilippo syndrome type B. *J Neurosci Res*. 93(3):424-32.

[27] Saitoh S. 2009. Chaperones and transport proteins regulate TLR4 trafficking and activation. *Immunobiology*. 214(7):594-600.

[28] Aflaki E, Moaven N, Borger DK, Lopez G, Westbroek W, Chae JJ, Marugan J, Patnaik S, Maniwang E, Gonzalez AN, Sidransky E. 2015. Lysosomal storage and impaired autophagy lead to inflammasome activation in Gaucher macrophages. *Aging Cell*. doi: 10.1111/acel.12409.

[29] Nair S, Boddupalli CS, Verma R, Liu J, Yang R, Pastores GM, Mistry PK, Dhodapkar MV. 2015. Type II NKT-TFH cells against Gaucher lipids regulate B-cell immunity and inflammation. *Blood*. 125(8):1256-71.

[30] Vidal-Donet JM, Cárcel-Trullols J, Casanova B, Aguado C, Knecht E. 2013. Alterations in ROS activity and lysosomal pH account for distinct patterns of macroautophagy in LINCL and JNCL fibroblasts. *PLoS One*. 8(2):e55526.

[31] Smith KR, Dahl HH, Canafoglia L, Andermann E, Damiano J, Morbin M, Bruni AC, Giaccone G, Cossette P, Saftig P, Grötzinger J, Schwake M, Andermann F, Staropoli JF, Sims KB, Mole SE, Franceschetti S, Alexander NA, Cooper JD, Chapman HA, Carpenter S, Berkovic SF, Bahlo M. 2013. Cathepsin F mutations cause Type B Kufs disease, an adult-onset neuronal ceroid lipofuscinosis. *Hum Mol Genet*. 22(7):1417-23.

[32] Tang CH, Lee JW, Galvez MG, Robillard L, Mole SE, Chapman HA. 2006. Murine cathepsin F deficiency causes neuronal lipofuscinosis and late-onset neurological disease. *Mol Cell Biol*. 26(6):2309-16.

[33] Murakawa T, Yamaguchi O, Hashimoto A, Hikoso S, Takeda T, Oka T, Yasui H, Ueda H, Akazawa Y, Nakayama H, Taneike M, Misaka T, Omiya S, Shah AM, Yamamoto A, Nishida K, Ohsumi Y, Okamoto K, Sakata Y, Otsu K. 2015 Bcl-2-like protein 13 is a mammalian Atg32

homologue that mediates mitophagy and mitochondrial fragmentation. *Nat Commun.* 6:7527.

[34] de Pablo-Latorre R, Saide A, Polishhuck EV, Nusco E, Fraldi A, Ballabio A. 2012. Impaired parkin-mediated mitochondrial targeting to autophagosomes differentially contributes to tissue pathology in lysosomal storage diseases. *Hum. Mol. Genet.* 21:1770-81.

[35] Osellame LD, Rahim AA, Hargreaves IP, Gegg ME, Richard-Londt A, Brandner S, Waddington SN, Schapira AH, Duchen MR. 2013. Mitochondria and quality control defects in a mouse model of Gaucher disease–links to Parkinson's disease. *Cell. Metab.* 17:941-53.

[36] Lim JA, Li L, Raben N. 2014. Pompe disease: from pathophysiology to therapy and back again. *Front Aging Neurosci.* 6:177.

[37] Li X, Gulbins E, Zhang Y. 2012. Oxidative stress triggers Ca-dependent lysosome trafficking and activation of acid sphingomyelinase. *Cell Physiol Biochem.* 30(4):815-26.

[38] Pelled D, Trajkovic-Bodennec S, Lloyd-Evans E, Sidransky E, Schiffmann R, Futerman AH. 2005. Enhanced calcium release in the acute neuronopathic form of Gaucher disease. *Neurobiol Dis.* 18(1): 83-8.

[39] Ginzburg L, Li SC, Li YT, Futerman AH. 2008. An exposed carboxyl group on sialic acid is essential for gangliosides to inhibit calcium uptake via the sarco/endoplasmic reticulum $Ca^{2+-}$ATPase: relevance to gangliosidoses. *J Neurochem.* 104(1):140-6.

[40] Ginzburg L, Futerman AH. 2005. Defective calcium homeostasis in the cerebellum in a mouse model of Niemann-Pick A disease. *J Neurochem.* 95(6):1619-28.

[41] Sano R, Annunziata I, Patterson A, Moshiach S, Gomero E, Opferman J, Forte M, d'Azzo A. 2009. $G_{M1}$-ganglioside accumulation at the mitochondria-associated ER membranes links ER stress to $Ca2^{+}$-dependent mitochondrial apoptosis. *Mol Cell.* 36(3):500-11.

[42] Chandrachud U, Walker MW, Simas AM, Heetveld S, Petcherski A, Klein M, Oh H, Wolf P, Zhao WN, Norton S, Haggarty SJ, Lloyd-Evans E, Cotman SL. 2015. Unbiased cell-based screening in a neuronal cell model of Batten disease highlights an interaction between $Ca^{2+}$ homeostasis, autophagy, and CLN3 Protein Function. *J Biol Chem.* 290(23):14361-80.

[43] Borbon IA, Hillman Z, Duran E Jr, Kiela PR, Frautschy SA, Erickson RP. 2012. Lack of efficacy of curcumin on neurodegeneration in the

mouse model of Niemann-Pick C1. *Pharmacol Biochem Behav.* 101(1):125-31.

[44] Cao Q, Zhong XZ, Zou Y, Zhang Z, Toro L, Dong XP. 2015. BK Channels alleviate lysosomal storage diseases by providing positive feedback regulation of lysosomal $Ca2^+$ release. *Dev Cell.* 33(4):427-41.

[45] Abou-Ghali M, Stiban J. 2015. Regulation of ceramide channel formation and disassembly: Insights on the initiation of apoptosis. *Saudi J Biol Sci.* 22(6):760-772.

[46] Bartsch U, Galliciotti G, Jofre GF, Jankowiak W, Hagel C, Braulke T. 2013. Apoptotic photoreceptor loss and altered expression of lysosomal proteins in the nclf mouse model of neuronal ceroid lipofuscinosis. *Invest Ophthalmol Vis Sci.* 54(10):6952-9.

[47] de Almagro MC, Vucic D. 2015. Necroptosis: Pathway diversity and characteristics. *Semin Cell Dev Biol.* 39:56-62.

[48] Vitner EB, Salomon R, Farfel-Becker T, Meshcheriakova A, Ali M, Klein AD, Platt FM, Cox TM, Futerman AH. 2014. RIPK3 as a potential therapeutic target for Gaucher's disease. *Nat Med.* 20(2):204-8.

[49] Lipton P. 2013. Lysosomal membrane permeabilization as a key player in brain ischemic cell death: a "lysosomocentric" hypothesis for ischemic brain damage. *Transl Stroke Res.* 4(6):672-84.

[50] Zeidan YH, Hannun YA. 2010. The acid sphingomyelinase/ceramide pathway: biomedical significance and mechanisms of regulation. *Curr Mol Med.* 10(5):454-66.

[51] Dattilo S, Mancuso C, Koverech G, Di Mauro P, Ontario ML, Petralia CC, Petralia A, Maiolino L, Serra A, Calabrese EJ, Calabrese V. 2015. Heat shock proteins and hormesis in the diagnosis and treatment of neurodegenerative diseases. *Immun Ageing.* 12:20.

[52] Cobb CA, Cole MP. 2015. Oxidative and nitrative stress in neurodegeneration. *Neurobiol Dis.* S0969-9961(15)00177-1.

[53] Shichiri M. 2014. The role of lipid peroxidation in neurological disorders. *J Clin Biochem Nutr.* 54(3):151-60.

[54] Wei H, Kim SJ, Zhang Z, Tsai PC, Wisniewski KE, Mukherjee AB. 2008. ER and oxidative stresses are common mediators of apoptosis in both neurodegenerative and non-neurodegenerative lysosomal storage disorders and are alleviated by chemical chaperones. *Hum Mol Genet.* 17(4):469-77.

*Chapter 3*

# Therapeutic and Preventive Options

## 3.1. Treatment Strategies

Directed commercially-available treatments for LSDs are focused on either 1) *enzyme replacement therapy* (ERT): the provision of exogenous recombinant protein, as a substitute for absent or deficient activity of the endogenous enzyme; or 2) *substrate reduction therapy* (SRT): the partial inhibition of substrate (precursor) synthesis by small molecular agents, to achieve intracellular metabolic homeostasis in a setting of reduced enzyme activity (*see* Figure 3.1). Prior to the availability of these pharmacologic options, bone marrow/hematopoietic stem cell transplantation (BMT/HSCT); i.e., cellular replacement therapy, had been performed in patients with various LSDs, and these procedures continue to be the primary therapeutic option for selected disorders, such as MPS-I (Hurler syndrome) and Krabbe disease (globoid cell leukodystrophy). Moreover, organ transplantation had been undertaken in patients with end-organ failure; e.g., kidney transplantation for patients with Fabry disease[24] and end-stage renal failure.

[24] Fabry disease is an X-linked LSD, caused by deficiency of the enzyme α-galactosidase A, associated with accumulation of the glycosphingolipid globotriaosylceramide (GL-3). Clinical manifestations include acrospaerethia, hearing loss, and hypohydrosis. Major sources of morbidity include renal failure, cardiomyopathy, arrhythmias and cerebrovascular disease (stroke).

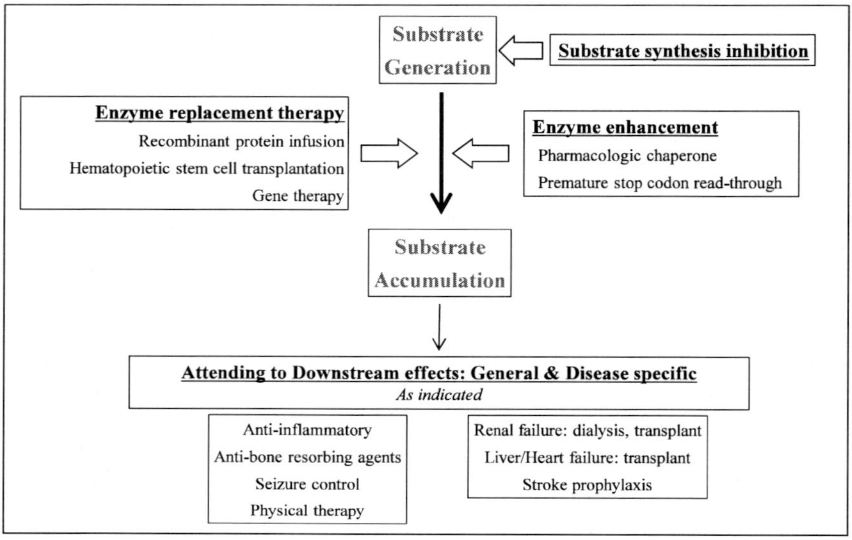


Figure 3.1. Therapeutic approaches for LSDs.

With the introduction of several therapeutic options, there is a need to define the full extent of clinical benefit from each drug; this is an aspect of management confounded by the lack of full knowledge regarding determinants of therapeutic outcome and the limited range of prescribed dose/frequency regimens. A practical issue relates to most patients having a significant disease burden by the time diagnosis is confirmed and treatment initiated. It has been suggested the latter concern may be addressed by targeted investigation of high-risk populations, and the expansion of current newborn screening programs to include certain LSDs.

Until recently, there has been a paucity of studies focusing on systematic evaluation of the natural history of specific lysosomal storage diseases; i.e., detailed examination of the pattern and severity of disease expression. There is also limited understanding of factors that may influence disease course. The availability of treatment for certain disorders has changed this state of affairs, with several efforts directed at appraising treatment benefits. Guidelines for the initiation and discontinuation of therapy are increasingly becoming available. Meanwhile, there are active investigations of biomarkers that may be useful in assessment of disease burden and that can potentially be incorporated in monitoring of the effects of treatment, in the hope of reducing or eliminating the need for invasive procedures, and perhaps aid with optimizing treatment regimens.

At present, transformative therapies for CNS-related complications do not exist, but there are on-going clinical trials to address this matter. Furthermore, it remains likely that existing therapies will not rectify all aspects of any given disease. In this instance, we may be confronted with emergent complications from partial cures; for which experience will be limited. Thus, vigilance and regular monitoring of treated patients will be essential; currently a voluntary effort is facilitated by various companies thorugh sponsored registry programs. Given the broad range of cell types and organs/systems involved, and the multiplicity of implicated disease pathways, combination therapies in due course may be required to attain the best clinical outcome. A comprehensive treatment approach may necessitate the use of adjunctive agents.

## a. Biologic, Cellular/Enzyme Replacement Therapy

The feasibility of treatment for the LSDs, initially involving cellular approaches (BMT) and subsequently by ERT (with the development of a means for industrial scale production of recombinant enzymes) came about following recognition of the phenomenon of metabolic 'cross-correction'. Essentially, in mixed skin fibroblast cultures it was observed that unaffected cells secreted a certain amount of lysosomal enzymes (the 'corrective factor'), which were captured by receptors (i.e., mannose-6-phosphate receptors) on the surface of affected cells, and subsequently internalized and directed to the lysosome; thereby restoring enzyme activity in affected cells and promoting the reduction of storage material within [1]. It had been anticipated correction of the underlying cellular defect would lead to clinical benefit, which has been realized to a certain extent. However, the experience to date has shown there are limitations to what can be achieved for some patients, and that these therapies do not represent a cure, as a 'burden' can be imposed by residual disease and associated complications. Furthermore, with ERT, there is a need for life-long infusions.

### *a.1. Hematopoietic Stem Cell (HSCT)/Bone Marrow Transplantation (BMT)*

With HSCT, donor-derived monocytes transmigrate through the blood brain barrier, enabling CNS access and ultimately the replacement of resident affected microglia by healthy cells. Thus, modification of CNS manifestations may be achieved, in conjunction with systemic responses.

Although HSCT has altered disease course, by preserving cognitive development in patients with Hurler syndrome (MPS-I), there has been no significant impact on the skeletal complications, which continues to influence quality of life among affected post-transplant cases [2]. Indeed, in most orthopaedic interventions are undertaken to address bone-related problems and bring relief from pain and preserve patient mobility.

Among those with infantile Krabbe disease, HSCT has led to increased survival [3]; however, there is evidence of gross motor deficits and associated ambulatory problems, noted in post-transplant patients past 2 years of age. The limited experience with HSCT in patients with NPC2 (a soluble non-enzymatic protein) suggests there may be benefits [4].

With HSCT there can be potential failure of full engraftment, and there are several procedure-related risks (e.g., graft *versus* host disease) including death. Early diagnosis, enabling early intervention is a key to optimal outcomes, and ideally, donor cells should be obtained from a non-carrier individual. The increasing use of cord blood has partly addressed issues related to lack of a donor pool and tissue histocompatibility.

The basis for the lack of efficacy of HSCT in the treatment of other LSDs associated with deficiency of a soluble enzyme (e.g., Hunter syndrome, Sanfilippo syndrome) is not understood. Recent studies in the mouse model of MPS-I have shown that excess overly-sulfated extracellular heparan sulfate binds and sequesters CXCL12[25], limiting hematopoietic migration and providing a potential mechanism for the limited scope of HSCT in Hurler disease, particularly on the bone-related features [5].

Currently, there are on-going studies in patients with Hurler syndrome aimed at evaluating the potential benefit of enzyme therapy prior to transplantation and through the period until full engraftment is established. It is hoped that this combined approach (HSCT + ERT) will lead to improved

[25] CXCL12, more commonly referred to as stromal-derived factor-1 (SF-1), acts as a chemo-attractant for a variety of adult stem cells including mesenchymal stem cells, hematopoietic stem cells, neural progenitor cells, and endothelial progenitor cells.

outcomes in these patients, as inferred from studies in the mouse model [6]. Increased overall well-being may also be achieved sooner, with a combined approached; although this needs to be formally examined. The impact of anitbodies against recombinant enzyme, potentially cross-reacting with donor cell-released enzyme also needs scrutiny.

### a.1.1. Mesenchymal/Stromal Stem Cells (MSC) as Donor Material

MSCs are deemed a developmentally-advantageous cell type with translational potential, and may be an additional transplant resource.

In the cystinosis (CTNS)[26] mouse model, infusion of human MSCs (derived from amniotic fluid or bone marrow) reversed the renal damage usually seen in this condition [7]. Moreover, *in vitro* co-culture studies (involving CTNS mutant fibroblasts *or* proximal tubular cells from cystinosis patients *and* donor wild type cells) revealed reduced pathologic cystine accumulation, attributed to the release into the culture medium of stem cell microvesicles containing wildtype cystinosin protein and CTNS mRNA [7].

In Purkinje neurons obtained from the NPC1 mouse model, bone marrow (BM) derived MSCs promoted survival, by correcting the altered calcium homeostasis and restoring the sphingolipid imbalance (as evidenced by increased sphingosine-1-phosphate and decreased sphingosine levels) [8]. As a consequence, there is inhibition of apoptosis pathways (mediated via activation of the ERK/RSK and downstream antiapoptotic signalling cascades). Additional beneficial effects may have resulted from the release of bioactive trophic factors by BM-MSCs.

In the *twitcher* mouse model of Krabbe disease[27], intracerebroventricular administration of MSCs on postnatal day 3-4 led to a significant increase in lifespan [9]. Body weight and motor function were improved in treated mice,

---

[26] Cystinosis is caused by mutations in the the lysosomal cystine transporter cystinosin (CTNS), resulting in the accumulation of cystine in the lysosomes of cells throughout the body and deregulation of endocytosis, the trafficking of intracellular vesicles and related cell signalling processes. Patients with the nephropathic subtype present with renal Fanconi syndrome, characterized by polyuria, proteinuria and urinary loss of various solutes. Subsequently, extrarenal complications become apparent, and decline of kidney function leads ultimately to the development of renal failure.

[27] Krabbe disease is an inherited demyelinating disorder characterized by deficiency of the enzyme β-galactosylceramidase, with consequent lysosomal psychosine accumulation and loss of myelin-forming cells. The *twitcher* mouse is a natural model of Krabbe disease bearing a spontaneous premature stop codon (p.W339X) in the cognate gene.

when compared with untreated controls. It was felt the stem cells mediated some of these benefits through an anti-inflammatory mechanism, because the expression of numerous pro-inflammatory markers was downregulated at both transcriptional and translational levels; associated with a marked decrease in the levels of macrophage infiltration and microglial activation [10].

In the MPS VII (Sly syndrome) mouse model, human umbilical MSCs have been transplanted into the corneal stroma. Subsequent evaluation revealed restoration of the dendritic and hexagonal morphology of host keratocytes and endothelial cells, respectively [11]. *In vivo* confocal microscopy revealed a reduction of the corneal haze, associated with a decrease in glycosaminoglycan (GAG) content, and both lysosomal number and size. *In vitro* co-culture assays (of skin fibroblasts isolated from MPS VII mice *and* wild type MSC) demonstrated that neutral vesicles released by the donor cells were taken up by affected fibroblasts and fused with the acidic lysosomes [11]. Also, these studies indicated transplanted MSCs participated in extracellular GAG turnover and enabled the host keratocytes to catabolize accumulated GAG products.

There is interest in ways to enhance MSC migration to relevant tissue sites and boost its effects, with studies focussing on the role of the chemokine receptor CXCR4 and its ligand SDF-1 (CXCL12). Investigations have shown that constitutive endocytosis is implicated in the regulation of CXCR4 membrane expression, which may be exploited as a means of enhancing the migration of systemically-transplanted cells by pharmacologic approaches [12]. For the MPS disorders, this approach may lead to improved skeletal outcomes, but requires further studies.

### *a.2. Enzyme Replacement Therapy*

Several recombinant proteins are now available for administration to patients with certain LSDs (Table 3.1). Prior to the conduct of clinical trials in human subjects, pre-clinical studies in animal models of disease, primarily affected mice generated by recombinant genetic techniques and in some cases dogs (e.g., canine model for MPS-I), were performed to establish ‘proof of therapeutic principle’. Exceptionally, trials for the first ERT product for an LSD (i.e., β-glucosidase used in the treatment of Gaucher disease) was initiated directly in affected individuals, as a suitable animal model had not been available during the course of drug development [13]. Moreover, prior to the availability of a recombinant formulation, the enzyme preparation given to patients had been purified from human placenta; modified to expose α-mannosyl residues by sequential deglycosylation of the glycoprotein hydrolase.

In an earlier era, there were attempts to use enzyme preparations purified from human tissue and other sources but these had been unsuccessful; for various different reasons, including the lack of sufficient quantities of the purified protein for regular administration. Moreover, in the case of Gaucher disease it was ultimately realized the purified enzyme had to be modified to expose the α-mannosyl residues, to target relevant cell types (i.e., cells of monocyte/macrophage lineage). As noted in Chapter 1, it was known that β-glucosidase did not rely, as with most lysosomal enzymes do, on M6P residues for cellular internalization.

**Table 3.1. Recombinant enzyme therapy for LSDs: Formulations**

| | |
|---|---|
| Imiglucerae (Genzyme\Sanofi)<br>Velaglucerase (Shire)<br>Taliglucerase (Protalix) | Gaucher disease |
| Agalsidase alfa (Shire)<br>Agalsidase beta (Genzyme\Sanofi) | Fabry disease |
| Sebilipase alfa (Syngeva\Alexion) | Lysosomal acid lipase deficiency, Wollman disease, Cholesterol ester storage disease |
| Laronidase (Biomarin\Genzyme) | Mucopolysaccharidosis I |
| Idursulfase (Shire) | Mucopolysaccharidosis II |
| Elosulfase (Biomarin) | Mucopolysaccharidosis IVA |
| Galsulfase (Biomarin) | Mucopolysaccharidosis VI |
| Myozyme (Genzyme\Sanofi) | Pompe disease, acid maltase deficiency |
| Beta-glucuronidase (rhGUS); investigational (Ultragenics) | Mucopolysaccharidosis VII |

Assessments of response to ERT have focused mainly on clearance of the accumulated substrate in plasma and\or tissues and corresponding clinical changes (such as improvements in blood counts, increased physical endurance), while data on increased survival and impact on patients' physical and functional well-being remain to be more fully delineated.

Apart from demonstration of reduced substrate storage, investigations are also unravelling potentially beneficial changes in biomarker profiles, following the administration of targeted treatments. For instance, direct molecular profiling from blood samples of patients with Fabry disease, before and after ERT, was undertaken to assess immune/inflammation and growth factor-related pathways. Analysis revealed that oxidative phosphorylation pathway-related genes were downregulated under treatment, which suggested a role in protection of proteins from oxidative damage [14]. Also found was increased levels of various markers: TINAGL1, DAAM2, CDK5R1 and MYO5B, potentially linked with amelioration of clinical manifestations; but this requires more through scrutiny.

In clinical practice, regular infusions of the cognate recombinant enzyme have been shown to alter the natural history of the corresponding LSD (Table 3.2), although treatment of symptomatic patients leaves much to be desired.

**Table 3.2. Recombinant enzyme therapy for LSDs: Outcomes**

| | |
|---|---|
| Gaucher disease | Improved blood counts, reduction of hepatosplenomegaly, improved bone density, prevention of bone related complications (in early treated cases) |
| Fabry disease | Partially mitigates neuropathic pain and gastrointestinal problems, modifies course of renal disease in mild to moderate CKD* (in the absence of significant proteinuria); stabilization or reduction of left ventricular hypertrophy (in the absence of fibrosis); but does not appear to alter the incidence of primary or secondary strokes |
| Lysosomal acid lipase deficiency | Reduction in aminotransferase levels and liver volume, and abatement of dyslipidemia (children and adults) |
| Mucopolysaccharidosis I, II, IVA, VI | Reduced urinary GAG+ excretion, reduction of hepatosplenomegaly, improvement in FVC^, increased physical endurance, based on distance travelled in a timed (6-minute) walk test |
| Pompe disease | Reduction of cardiomegaly, improved lifespan and delay in the need for or relief from ventilator support (infantile cases); delay in progression of muscle weakness, based on distance travelled in a timed walk test (late-onset case) |

*CKD, chronic kidney disease; ^FVC, forced vital capacity; +GAG, glycosaminoglycans.

Pre-existing pathology is one of several determinants of outcome. As an example, in patients with Fabry disease, myocardial fibrotic changes are associated with persistent cardiomyopathy and risk of malignant ventricular arrhythmias, which can lead to sudden death [15]. In these patients, serial monitoring is important to identify those at grave risk, as reduction of propensity for sudden cardiac death may be achieved by the timely placement of an intracardiac pacing/defibrillator device. Interestingly, a recent report has found risk for cardiac-related complications to be similar among patients with cardiac-predominant mutations (associated with residual enzyme activity) *and* those with Fabry disease associated with classic mutations (which in most cases manifest with renal involvement among males and in some female relatives) [16]. Interestingly, although gentype was not predictive of outcome (i.e., cardiac-related complications) QRS duration (HR 1.03; CI 1.0-1.05; p = 0.02) on an electrocardiogram was informative.

In Pompe disease, neuropathological investigations have revealed changes in respiratory motor neurons and limb muscle neuromuscular junctions as factors that contribute to muscle weakness. Thus, clearance of muscle glycogen storage may not be sufficient to achieve a full clinical response, when tissue damage has occurred before treatment has been initiated and/or when disease involves affected sites that may not be fully accessed by intravenous infusions of the recombinant enzyme [17].

### a.2.1. Antibodies to the Infused Enzyme

Varying proportions of patients on ERT have developed antibodies to the infused recombinant enzyme, although in most cases the presence of circulating antibodies does not abrogate benefits accrued from treatment [18]. However, in patients with infantile-onset Pompe disease antibodies that develop against the drug significantly reduced its efficacy, and immunomodulatory regimens have been developed to address this problem [19]; which appear to work best when given to patients assessed as CRIM-negative at baseline, and anti-rejection medications are initiated concurrently with enzyme therapy. Recent experience suggests this may also be the case in some patients with Fabry disease treated with recombinant enzyme (agalsidase), although there are no descriptions of such patients being given immunomodulatory agents concomittantly.

Enzyme therapy is generally well tolerated, and adverse events are often mitigated by a slower rate of infusion and the use of a more dilute solution. In some patients, infusion related adverse events may be ameliorated by the use of premedication, primarily a combination of an anti-pyretic and an antihistamine, and occasionally the use of steroids. The relatively short half-life of the enzyme in plasma may limit drug exposure to circulating antibodies, which may reduce the formation of immune complexes and the overall negative effects of antidrug antibodies. In most treated patients who have sero-converted (i.e., developed antibodies against the enzyme), antibody-titers appear to decrease over time.

An observation of interest, in relation to factors besides anti-enzyme antibodies which may influence outcome is the finding from cell-based experiments which revealed propranolol reduced the uptake of rhGAA (myozyme) into Pompe (α-glucosidase-deficient) fibroblasts and induced intracellular accumulation of glycoproteins in a dose related manner [20]. On the other hand, albuterol, which enhances the expression of cation-independent M6P receptor, has been shown to enhance muscle glycogen clearance in Pompe mice receiving enzyme therapy [21]. Further studies may clarify which additional drugs may be necessary or proscribed, according to their influence on enzyme delivery and uptake.

### a.2.2. The Blood-Brain-Barrier (BBB) Issue

Delivery of therapeutic proteins across the blood-brain-barrier (*see* Figure 3.2) remains a major challenge, when aiming for the correction of neurodegenerative diseases. In the case of LSDs, there is no substantive evidence that the integrity of the BBB is breached; indeed, none of the currently available recombinant enzymes administered intravenously alter ultimate neurologic prognosis in treated patients. Several approaches are under consideration to improve brain drug-delivery, including generation of chimeric enzymes that incorporates a specific protein ligand to facilitate uptake via transcytosis receptors (e.g., uptake through clathrin- or cell adhesion molecule-mediated mechanisms).

One study has reported improved delivery of acid sphingomyelinase (the enzyme deficient in Niemann-Pick A/B disease), modified for targeted delivery through integration of antibodies against intercellular adhesion molecule-1 (ICAM-1)[28] and the transferrin receptor (Tfr) [22].

There has been interest in the potential to increase drug levels within the CNS following intravenous infusions, using particulate delivery vehicles such

[28] Enzymes targeted through ICAM-1 (an immunoglobulin-like transmembrane glycoprotein expressed in most cells) involve cell-adhesion-mediated endocytosis; which by-passes the traditional route of clathrin-mediated endocytosis. It is believed the interaction of ICAM-1 with NHE-1 (sodium/proton exchanger protein-1) and signalling through the sphingomyelin/ceramide cascade results in the modification of the immediate plasma membrane and re-organization of the actin cytoskeleton, leading to the uptake of the relevant enzyme.

as colloidal nanoparticles (which can also incorporate sensing by means of pH tracking). Recombinant formulations of α-glucosidase (enzyme deficient in Pompe coupled to polymer nanocarriers (NCs; ~180 nm) coated with an antibody specific to ICAM-1, promoted enzyme uptake in a glycosylation-independent manner [23, 24].

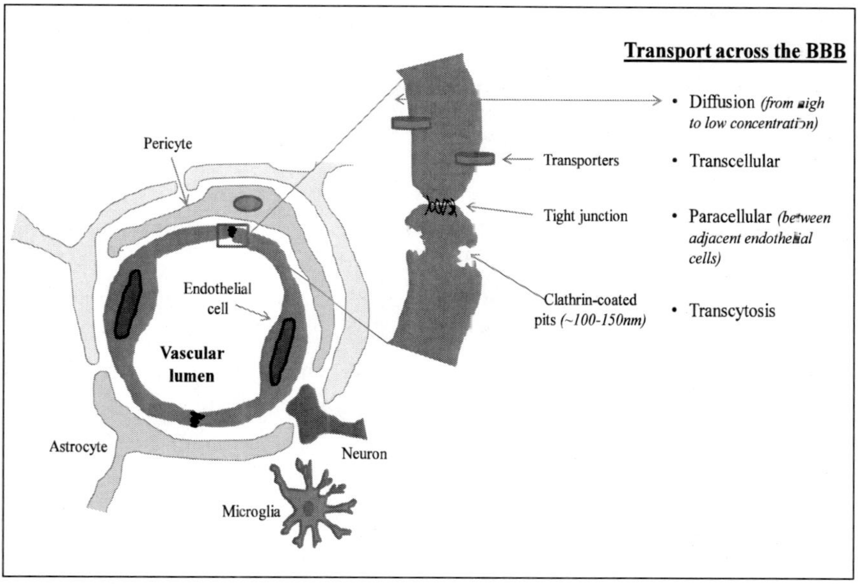


Figure 3.2. Blood-brain-barrier and transport processes.

### a.2.3. Fusion Proteins

Beyond the issue of the blood-brain-barrier, there is also the added multiplicity of affected cell types, which may necessitate different methods of targeting the therapeutic proteins to achieve an optimal outcome usin g mixed formulations.

Alternative means for intracellular delivery of the exogenous enzyme (or the protein secreted from transduced cells, *see following section on Gene therapy*) that does not rely on glycosyl-receptors is being explored. This approach involves the production of chimeric proteins which incorporate a targeting section, such as insulin-like growth factor II (which binds to a different domain of the M6P receptor) [25]. Other such proteins contain the receptor-associated protein RAP, which targets the LDL-R family of receptors

[26]. Both of these forms of fusion proteins are internalized via clathrin-dependent mechanisms.

Besides exploiting receptor-mediated endocytosis, fusion proteins that contain a transduction domain such as peptides derived from the HIV transcription factor TAT, may improve on delivery by charge-dependent binding to the plasma membrane [27]. Such modification has been undertaken with arlsulfatase A (enzyme deficient in metachromatic leukodystrophy). Internalization of the modified enzyme can then occur via passive uptake within endocytic vesicles or direct penetration through the plasmalemma.

### a.2.4. Further Considerations

Enzyme therapy for several LSDs has been beneficial, with the best outcome observed in treated patients with GD type 1. For those conditions associated with primary CNS involvement (e.g., severe Hunter and Hurler syndromes) and/or neuromuscular disease (e.g., Pompe), ultimately patients may show disease progression and reach a state of severe debility, including advanced respiratory insufficiency. In these cases, there is the difficult decision which has to be made regarding on-going enzyme therapy, when it becomes clear that such an approach may be futile. Measures to relieve pain and suffering must be a focus, with the goal of sustaining quality of life and preserving patient dignity. End of life care and involvement of the palliative team to facilitate the process of communicating with relevant parties and coordinating management of patients to the point of death and beyond (i.e., grieving and bereavement) becomes critical.

## b. Pharmacologic/Small Molecule Therapies

Non-biologic drugs for the treatment of LSDs include chemical agents that either: a) inhibit substrate (precursor) synthesis, or b) act as pharmacologic chaperones. The latter approach entails the restoration of residual enzyme activity above a threshold which is sufficient to enable on-going substrate clearance; this is realized by rescuing the mutant protein from premature degradation, and enabling the transit of the mutant enzyme to the lysosome.

The possibility that energy imbalance and a disturbance of intermediary metabolism may be a contributory disease event in certain LSDs has led to the suggestion that substrate synthesis inhibitors may also have a secondary role in restoring cellular homeostasis, by reducing the demand for raw materials necessary for *de novo* synthesis of stored substrates.

A third option involves drugs that promote transcriptional read-through, in cases wherein the causal mutation (i.e., null alleles) results in premature termination of the nascent protein's synthesis. Other small molecule therapies, aimed at correcting pathology and whose action is not related to the primary clearance of substrate or correction of the cognate protein defect are covered in a latter section (on *Adjunctive therapies*).

Potential advantages of small molecule therapies include the absence of antibody formation against the administered chemical drug and selection of a formulation that can be given orally (in contrast to intravenous administration, as undertaken with ERT). Moreover, chemical agents may have broader biodistribution, including deep tissues that may not be accessible to recombinant protein therapies (which is dependent on receptor medicated uptake). Moreover, it would be feasible to alter side-chains of a chemical drug to generate a preparation with an optimal safety and efficacy profile. On the other hand, there may be off-target effects, and potential for interaction with other drugs that the patient may be on.

### *b.1. Substrate Synthesis Inhibition*

Miglustat (*N-butyldeoxynojirimycin*), an alkylated iminosugar, was the first oral agent shown to have clinical efficacy and was relatively safe when used in the treatment of Gaucher disease type 1 in adult patients deemed not suitable for ERT [28]. It has also been shown to have some beneficial effects in a few patients with Niemann-Pick type C disease [29], for which it has gained regulatory approval in Europe.

A more potent formulation, Eliglustat, has recently been introduced into clinical practice for adult patients with type 1 GD following demonstration of its safety and efficacy in several clinical trials; these studies involved different groups of patients, including those naïve to treatment and those who had previously been on enzyme therapy ('switched' group) [30, 31]. Thus far, there are no emergent adverse effects that would halt use of the drug, and an increasing number of patients may show a preference for oral *versus* intravenous therapy. Clinical trials remain to to be undertaken in pediatric patients.

### b.2. Pharmacologic Chaperone Rescue

A mutation which results in the misfolding of the emerging protein in the endoplasmic reticulum (ER) is recognized by the ER-quality control system (ER-associated degradation, ERAD) and prematurely degraded, usually via the ubiquitin-proteasome pathways. Specific proteins, such as the inositol-requiring enzyme-1 (IRE-1), monitor the ER for the balance between misfolded protein load and capacity to deal with it; which involves the possibility of salvaging the protein through mobilization of endogenous chaperones, or facilitating its clearance by means of ERAD pathways and subsequent diversion of damaged protein to the ubiquitin-proteasomal system [32]. Besides facilitating the folding of nascent polypeptide chains, chaperones facilitate protein translocation across various cellular compartments, protect against protein aggregation, and when required promote the assembly/ disassembly of multiprotein complexes.

In cases wherein the causal mutations destabilize the protein's native structure but do not directly impair its catalytic activity, there may be a possibility to rescue the misfolded protein. Screening studies, which have relied primarily on exposure of affected cells in culture to a candidate drug, have led to the identification of small molecule agents (referred to as pharmacologic chaperones) that selectively bind to and stabilize the target protein, permitting its trafficking to the lysosome. An upshot is the restoration (so called 'enhancement') of intralysosomal (residual) enzyme activity, which may be sufficient to facilitate substrate clearance.

As noted, this strategy is applicable in cases wherein the underlying mutation does *not* (1) inactive the enzyme's activity; which occurs with a mutation within the active site, or (2) lead to rapid degradation of the mRNA (i.e., subject to non-sense mediated decay, which prevents generation of the related protein), or (c) a truncated protein product (e.g., deletion mutations). As such, putative agents may be useful only for a subset of patients, primarily those with so-called permissive (missense) mutations. Moreover, given broad heterogeneity in causal mutations the increase in residual enzyme activity can be variable, and it might be difficult to ascertain – *a priori* - the exact relationship between the observed increased activity *in vitro* (when measured in patient's fibroblasts or lymphoblasts), and anticipated substrate clearance *in vivo* and corresponding clinical response, if any.

The majority of pharmacologic chaperones which have been identified to date are reversible active site inhibitors that are displaced from the mutant enzyme within the low pH of the lysosome and that enzyme's greater affinity for its natural substrate.

The iminosugar, 1-deoxygalactonojirimycin (migalastat hydrochloride), is an analog of the terminal galactose of GL-3 (the primary lipid which accumulates in Fabry disease). Migalastat reversibly binds and stabilizes wild type and mutant forms of α-galactosidase A. Used as monotherapy, it has been shown to reduce the storage of GL-3 *in vitro* and *in vivo [33]*. Preliminary data suggests a decrease in left ventricular mass occurs in migalastat-treated patients, when compared with those on placebo. Studies have also shown that migalastat in combination with agalsidase may be expected to enhance the pharmacokinetics of agalsidase in plasma, and potentially lead to increased cellular levels of the enzyme in disease-relevant tissues [34]. Further studies are required to ascertain the clinical benefit of migalastat monotherapy, and when used in combination with ERT.

### *b.3. Agents that Promote a Read-through of Premature Stop Codons*

Nonsense and frameshift mutations that generate premature termination codons (PTCs) account for approximately a third of deleterious alleles leading to an LSD. Nonsense-mediated mRNA decay (NMD) is a regulatory pathway that functions to degrade transcripts containing PTCs; which in the case of LSDs leads to loss of hydrolytic capacity within lysosomes and consequent substrate storage.

Certain drugs, such as aminoglycosides and PTC124 (ataluren), have been found to promote the read-through of in-frame premature stop codons introduced by nonsense mutations, and thereby, enable the production of full-length proteins. It is likely that diverse drugs induce different salutary effects on nonsense mutations of specific genes. Some studies have suggested the mutation site may be a significant factor in determining the efficiency of pharmacological rescue. Moreover, studies have indicated inter-individual variability in the efficiency of NMD. Thus, the potential of these agents to effect a response will need close clinical investigation, to ascertain the subgroup of patients most likely to benefit.

A report has described the use of gentamicin and ataluren, to enhance stop-codon read-through and restore the production of full-length arylsulfatase B (ARSB, the enzyme deficient in MPS VI). These fibroblast-based studies examined drug effects on four different ARSB nonsense mutations (p.R315X, p.R327X, p.Q456X and p.Q503X) [35]. Interestingly, ataluren (but not gentamicin) increased the level of ARSB activity in three MPS VI patients' fibroblast cell lines, with enzyme activity levels in two of these noted to be significantly higher than in untreated cells; associated with a significant reduction of lysosomal size. The basis of this differential response, between drugs used and cell lines involved, is not known.

Similarly, the aminoglycoside NB84 restored α-L-iduronidase function via PTC suppression to reduce tissue GAG accumulation in the *Idua*(tm1Kmke) MPS I-Hurler mouse model, which carries a mutation homologous to the human *IDUA*-p.W402X mutation. Following a 28-week treatment period, there was a significant moderation of the disease in multiple tissues, including the brain, heart and bone [36]. Clinical trials with ataluren are currently being conducted in patients with MPS-I bearing null alleles (p.W402X; p.Q77X).

In infantile NCL (caused by mutations in *CLN1*), nonsense mutations account for 52.3% of disease-causing alleles, with a common mutation (p.R151X) described worldwide. In studies involving the affected mouse model incorporating the p.R151X mutation, administration of ataluren increased the protein level and activity of the relevant enzyme, palmitoyl-protein thioesterase 1 [37].

## c. Alternative Approaches to Facilitate Substrate Clearance, Through Action on Downstream Events

The cyclic oligosaccharide 2-hydroxypropyl-β-cyclodextrin (clycodextrin for short) is a solubilizing agent of lipophilic compounds; an excipient used to improve the stability and bioavailability of several drugs. Studies have indicated cyclodextrin may be a potential therapy for Niemann-Pick type C (NPC) disease.

Investigations involving the NPC mouse model revealed subcutaneous injection of cyclodextrin improved lifespan, associated with the prevention of liver injury and cholesterol sequestration [38]. The putative mechanism of action of cyclodextrin has not been fully elucidated; a relevant role may include its ability to extract cholesterol from the plasma membrane, which strongly influences the cholesterol content of intracellular membranes and enables correction of underlying signalling or trafficking problems. More recent studies in fibroblasts from a patient with late infantile NCL revealed cyclodextrin enhanced the autophagic clearance of ceroid lipopigment, mediated by the transcription factor TFEB [39]. As defects in autophagic flux have been shown in NPC, this observation may also be applicable for this condition and other LSDs, but this premise requires experimental demonstration.

Intravenous administration of cyclodextrin in two Japanese NPC patients was shown to be partially effective in improving hepatosplenomegaly and central nervous system dysfunction [40]. However, there was no apparent recovery of major neurological deficits in either patient. A separate study, involving a 12-year old NPC patient given cyclodextrin intrathecally (via lumbar puncture) described an improvement in vertical gaze [41]. Unfortunately, the child developed subclinical high frequency hearing loss that was deemed related to the study drug. Further investigations are required to ascertain the safety and efficacy of cyclodextrin, when given to patients with NPC, and the best means or route of drug delivery. Improved understanding of its mechanism of action may lead to identification of other candidate drugs with a wider safety margin.

Another drug, genistein (5,7-dihydroxy-3-(4-hydroxyphenyl)-4H-1-benzopyran-4-one), a flavone initially shown to inhibit the synthesis of glycosaminoglycans, has recently be shown to promote TFEB-mediated exocytosis [42]. The fate of exocytosed substrate in these instance, and the resultant functional/beneficial implications, if any, are unknown at this time.

## d. Adjunctive Therapies, Aimed at Correction of Associated Clinical Manifestations

Several aspects relating to pathogenesis in certain LSDs are not fully understood; examples include osteopenia in Gaucher disease (partly attributed to osteoclast activation), and cardiomyopathy in Fabry disease (which may be partly assigned to an intermediary substrate Lyso-Gb3, which has been shown to promote smooth muscle proliferation *in vitro*). Although enzyme therapy for the LSDs alters the rate of disease progression, certain drugs (and interventions) may be necessary to achieve an overall positive outcome. These may include the use of agents which modulate the immune response or other relevant pathways implicated in disease expression, that occur in parallel with substrate accumulation or as downstream events. For instance, in patients with

Fabry disease, the administration of angiotensin converting enzyme inhibitors (for its renoprotective properties), lipid-lowering drugs, and aspirin or antiplatelet-aggregating agents may reduce the risk of sentinel events, such as rapid progression to renal failure and embolic stroke [43].

Patients with Pompe disease are at risk for sleep disordered breathing (generally, when upright vital capacity (VC) is <60% of predicted value) and sustained nocturnal hypercapnia (generally, when upright VC is <40% of predicted) [44]. These patients benefit from continuous positive airway pressure (CPAP) ventilation. Furthermore, these patients are at risk for osteopenia and fractures, which is increased in those who are non-weight bearing and have muscle atrophy [45]. Optimized nutrition and vitamin D supplementation may be required to fully address this problem.

Additionally, patients with late-onset Pompe disease (LOPD) may benefit from endurance and resistance type exercises, which can promote increased muscle strength and performance. These workouts may also be associated with improvement in inspiratory and expiratory muscle strength. In conjunction, a low carbohydrate/high protein diet has been proposed as potentially helpful in preserving muscle mass [46]. A study from the pre-ERT era described an improvement or plateau in motor function score (based on the Walton & Gardner-Medwin Scale) in patients with LOPD on such a diet and exercise program.

Aberrant neuroimmune responses are believed to be an instrumental factor in certain neurodegenerative LSDs. Thus, there are on-going preclinical studies to examine the potential use of agents that can modulate immune responses (related to disease, as against those in response to enzyme administration or gene therapy), but none have been integrated into clinical practice, as yet. In the mouse model for juvenile Batten disease (NCL3) immunosuppression with mycophenolate mofetil altered disease course and severity [47]. The findings from this study provided the rationale to advance to a phase I clinical trial 'Cellcept for treatment of Juvenile NCL' (Clintrials.gov identifier NCT01 399047).

*Briefly, on combined pharmacologic treatments:* Triple combination therapy (using miglustat, curcumin and ibuprofen) was shown to have greater neuroprotective benefit in NPC1 mice, compared with single and dual therapies. Such a combined regimen has led to an increase in the time period that NPC1 mice maintained body weight and motor function, and it maximally delayed the onset of Purkinje cell loss [48]. Ibuprofen selectively reduced microglial activation, while curcumin[29] had no anti-inflammatory effects; indicating differential mechanisms of action for these two therapies that may have synergistic effects.

## e. Gene Therapy

As LSDs are caused primarily by a *loss of function* mutations in single recessive genes, they are viewed as prime candidates for gene therapy (GT). A major factor in the selection of disease target is the nature of the mutated protein (i.e., whether it is a soluble or membrane-bound protein). With regards to deficient enzymes, even a small increase in residual activity may be sufficient to alter the course of disease significantly, as evident from studies of the natural history of late-onset variants. Furthermore, there is the possibility of correcting non-transduced cells, through uptake of enzymes secreted by transformed cells. For instance, liver-directed GT may enable robust production and secretion of the cognate enzyme for distribution to peripheral tissues. Moreover, the use of liver-specific promoters may avoid immune responses by preventing transgene expression within antigen-presenting cells.

In some cases, the desired gene product may not be a deficient enzyme but a protein involved with substrate transport. In this regards, overexpression of recombinant human Rab9 fused with the herpes simplex virus VP22 protein fragment in NPC1 fibroblasts was found to lead to significant reduction in cellular free cholesterol levels [49]. The reduction in cellular free cholesterol was associated with correction of abnormal intracellular membrane trafficking of BODIPY-lactosylceramide; changes that may have therapeutic potential. As evident in this case, transport defects may be addressed through other routes; in cases wherein correction of the specific causal gene defect may not be feasible.

Pharmacologic approaches that influence gene expression or the stability of its product, are also under investigation. For example, it has been found that

[29] Curcumin is a major active polyphenol component, extracted from the rhizomes of Curcuma longa (Zingiberaceae). It has been reported to exert neuroprotective effects in several experimental models. Mechanistic studies have demonstrated that curcumin significantly restored the expression levels of heme oxygenase-1 and NAD(P)H:quinone oxidoreductase 1; ameliorating rotenone-induced neurotoxicity *in vivo*, via the phosphorylation of Akt and nuclear factor erythroid 2-related factor 2 (Nrf2).

histone deacetylase (HDAC)[30] inhibitors (e.g., vorinostat) that are effective against HDACs 1, 2, and 3 reduce cholesterol accumulation in fibroblasts derived from NPC1 patients. This finding is believed to result from the post-translational stabilization of the NPC1 protein, allowing it to be transported out of the endoplasmic reticulum and delivered to the lysosome [50]. Similarly, the use of proteasome inhibitors[31] (e.g., bortezomib) may be beneficial. Fibroblast from NPC1 patients exposed to bortezomib had partial recovery of mutant protein activity, associated with substantial reduction in free cholesterol levels [51]. Further studies will be required to ascertain the safety and efficacy of these agents in the treatment of patients with NPC1.

### *e.1. Viral Vectors*

Viral mediated gene therapy, in which a cDNA encoding wild type-protein is packaged into lentiviral or adeno-associated viral (AAV) particles, remains a promising therapeutic option. Early efforts examined the potential use of retroviral vectors. In patients with Gaucher disease, an initial attempt was uneventful and without adverse events; however, β-glucosidase gene expression was not sustained and thus, not established as curative [52].

Lentiviruses (LV) are enveloped single-stranded RNA viruses of the Retroviridae family. An advantage of LVs is their capacity for packaging: 10 kb in LV *versus* 4.8 kb in Adeno-associated viruses (AAVs). LVs also exhibit a low level of immunogenicity and in its capacity to initiate a systemic immune response; an important safety consideration, particularly if repeated administration becomes necessary [53]. LVs do not display tissue-specific tropism; however, they can be pseudotyped via alteration of envelope proteins, usually with the vesicular stomatitis glycoprotein. Transduction is limited to the site of injection, with no anterograde or retrograde transport; although

[30] Histone dacetylases (HDAC) are a group of enzymes that remove acetyl groups from histones and regulate gene expression. HDAC inhibitors interfere with HDAC activity and regulate biological events, such as cell cycle, differentiation and apoptosis.

[31] The ubiquitin-proteasome system (UPS) plays a central role in maintaining cellular homeostasis by controlling the apporpriate breakdown of key proteins, including those involved in cell cycle regulation, activation of transcription factors (for example, NF-κB) and the induction of apoptosis. The ubiquitin component marks proteins that need to be processed; whilst the proteasome module is a 26S structure which consists of the 19S regulator and the 20S central proteolytic core. Proteasome inhibitors are potentially useful drugs that can modulate immune response (when necessary), based on their ability to (a) inhibit the activation of nuclear factor NF-κB and transcriptional regulation of pro-inflammatory cytokine release, and/or (b) induce apoptosis of activated immune cells.

modification of the envelope to contain chimeric rabies glycoproteins results in significant retrograde trafficking. Nonetheless, the latter phenomenon does not compare to the trafficking efficacy of some of AAV serotypes.

LVs integrate into the host genome and allow the transgene to be expressed. Integration enables persistent gene expression in dividing cell populations. However, nonspecific integration, especially in areas that are actively replicating, could cause unintended serious consequences. To minimize or avoid insertional mutagenesis, non-integrating LV vectors which maintain episomal expression are currently under development. Inclusion of 'transcriptional insulators' may decrease the chance of activating bystander genes.

Adeno-associated viruses (AAV) are non-enveloped single-stranded DNA viruses from the Parvoviridae family. Qualities of recombinant AAVs that make them appealing as a gene therapy vector for neurodegenerative disorders include: 1) many serotypes derived from multiple host species, each presenting unique tropisms for different tissue types; e.g., AAV2 demonstrates natural tropism towards neurons over other cell types; 2) widespread distribution of the vector in the CNS via axonal transport; and 3) tropism for post-mitotic long-lived tissue [53]. Moreover, recombinant AAV remains predominantly episomal, reducing risk associated with integration into key genomic sites in host cells. Enduring episomal maintenance and expression in non-dividing cells precludes the need for constant dosing and consequential complications.

The main hurdle with AAV use is the induction of an immune response, which can be associated with small titres of neutralising antibodies. Most individuals harbour antibodies against AAV2, derived from naturally occurring prior exposure to these viruses. The presence of these antibodies elicits a humoral immune response, which can be a deterrent to achieving successful gene transfer. The degree of immune responses to AAV vectors is believed to differ based on the route of administration. Modulating immune response to protein product and/or the viral vector are critical in obtaining a successful outcome.

### e.1.1. Recent Preclinical and Clinical Studies (Listed in Table 3.3)

Infusion of hematopoietic stem cells (HSCs), obtained from three presymptomatic patients with metachromatic leukodystrophy (MLD) and transduced beforehand with a functional arylsulfatase A (*ARSA*) gene using a lentiviral vector, showed extensive and stable ARSA protein replacement.

High enzyme expression throughout hematopoietic lineages and in the cerebrospinal fluid was observed [54]. Follow-up revealed no detectable signs of disease activity or progression, 7 to 21 months beyond the predicted age of symptom onset.

An alternative approach, for which preclinical studies have been undertaken, involved the intracerebral administration of an AAVrh.10-h*ARSA* vector, coding for the human enzyme. Initial studies were conducted in MLD mice lacking *Arsa* gene expression. Subsequent experiments involved nonhuman primates (NHPs), given either the dose planned for patients adjusted to the brain volume ratio between child and NHP (1×dose, $1.1 \times 10^{11}$ viral genomes (vg)/hemisphere, unilateral or bilateral injection) *or* 5-fold this dose (5×dose, $5.5 \times 10^{11}$ vg/hemisphere, bilateral injection) [55]. Following administration of the lower dose, AAVrh.10-h*ARSA* vector was detected in a large part of the injected hemisphere, while ARSA enzyme activity exceeded the normal endogenous activity level by 14-31%. A neuroinflammatory process correlating with increased brain MRI T2 signals was absent or minimal on the lower dose, but observed by 90 days after administration of the higher dose. Antibody response to both AAVrh.10 and h*ARSA* was detected, without correlation with brain lesions. Thus, dose selection will also be an important factor in striking a balance between potential for benefit in relation to risk of adverse events.

**Table 3.3. Gene therapy clinical trials for neuropathic LSDs**

| Disorder | Phase | Vector | Route |
|---|---|---|---|
| LINCL | I | AAV2 | Intracranial |
| LINCL | I/II | AAVrh.10 | Intracranial |
| MLD | I/II | Lentivirus | HSCT |
| MLD | I | AAVrh.10 | Intracranial |
| MPS-IIIA | I | AAVrh.10 | Intracranial |
| MPS-I | I | Retrovirus | HSCT |
| MPS-II | I | Retrovirus | HSCT |
| MPS-VII | I | Lentivirus | HSCT |
| Galactosialidosis | I | scAAV8 | Intravenous |
| Tay-Sachs disease | I | AAV1 | Intravenous and intrathecal |

Four children (patients no. 1-3 ages, between 5.5 and 6 years; and patient no. 4 age, 2 years 8 months) with Mucopolysaccharidosis type IIIA (Sanfilippo syndrome type A) received intracerebral injections of an AAVrh.10 incorporating the cognate enzyme (sulfamidase, SGSH)-IRES and its activator (SUMF1) [56]. The therapeutic vector was delivered at a dose of $7.2 \times 10^{11}$ vg/patient simultaneously via 12 needles, as deposits of 60 μl over a period of 2 hr. [Target site: bilaterally, to the white matter anterior, medial, and posterior to the basal ganglia.] Immunosuppressive treatment (mycophenolate mofetil and tacrolimus) was initiated 15 days before surgery and maintained for 8 weeks (mycophenolate mofetil) or throughout follow-up (tacrolimus, with progressive dose reduction) to prevent rejection/elimination of transduced cells.

In the study just described, the procedure was well tolerated, and no adverse events related to the injected product were observed. Furthermore, there was no increase in the number of infectious events and no biological sign of toxicity related to the use of immunosuppressive drugs. All children were able to walk, but their cognitive abilities were abnormal and had declined (in patients no. 1-3) [56]. Patients no. 1-3 presented with brain atrophy prior to treatment, which was deemed to have stabilized in patients no. 1 and 3 but tended to increase in patients no. 2 and 4. Neuropsychological evaluations suggested a possible moderate improvement in behavior, attention, and sleep in patients no. 1-3. It was concluded the youngest patient had the most benefit. Thus, early treatment proffers the best scenario for a positive outcome.

Studies have also been conducted with AAV vector-mediated genetic modification of either skeletal muscle or liver in 2-month-old MPS-IIIA (sulfamidase deficient) mice. Intramuscular administration of AAV-*SGSH* failed to achieve significant therapeutic benefit, despite high levels of sulfamidase activity in muscle (which was not released into the circulation); whereas AAV8-mediated liver-directed gene transfer achieved high and sustained levels of circulating active enzyme [57]. In the latter case, there was complete clearance of lysosomal GAG accumulation in most somatic tissues. Remarkably, a 50% reduction of GAG accumulation was achieved throughout the entire brain of affected male mice, which correlated with a partial improvement of pathologic features of the cerebellum and cortex. Importantly, liver-directed gene transfer expanded the lifespan of treated MPS-IIIA males.

### *e.2. Non-Viral Gene Vectors for Therapeutic Protein Expression*

Synthetic 'vehicles' are being explored as means of modulating gene expression, as they tend to have lower immunogenicity than viral vectors and may have potential for a larger genetic payload and be easier to produce [58]. Cargo may range from DNA, mRNA, small interfering (si)RNA, microRNA or antisense oligonucleotides. For non-viral gene therapy approaches, naked plasmid DNA represents one of the most popular vector. Physical delivery strategies include electroporation, sonoporation or hydrodynamics-based techniques, and magnetofection. Entrapment of nucleic acids in nanoparticles may provide protection from endonuclease degradation and improve circulation time and ultimate tissue delivery.

Hydrodynamic delivery of *SGSH* (sulfamidase)-encoding pFAR4 (an antibiotic-free expression plasmid vector) into the liver of MPS-IIIA mice has been shown to lead to high serum levels of sulfamidase (the protein) that was efficiently taken up by neighbouring systemic organs, as shown by the reduction of GAG accumulation in several organs [59]. There was a similar reduction in brain GAG content, which occurred at early stages of the disease.

More recently, there has been growing interest in examining the potential of repairing disease-causing gene defects, through genome-editing systems, such as CRISPR-Cas. The later has been used to correct a disease mutation for an inborn of metabolism (*viz.*, hereditary tyrosinemia in adult mice) and shown to rescue the phenotype [60].

## 3.2. Prevention, Newborn and Target Population Screening, and Aspects Relating to Genetic Counselling

Newborn screening will be necessary for certain LSDs, to prevent or reduce the burden of devastating complications related to CNS and bone disease; for which early initiation of therapy will be critical. Early diagnosis will also enable genetic counselling regarding reproductive risks, so families can plan accordingly. Pre-implantation genetic testing and/or prenatal diagnosis has been undertaken by couples to manage risk. Early diagnosis may enable initiation of treatment in an oligosymptomatic patient who are at risk of disease progression.

The combined birth prevalence of LSDs ranges from 7.5 (in British Columbia) to 23.5 (United Arab Emirates, UAE) per 100,000 live births, with the sphingolipidoses noted as the most frequent disease category in most populations, followed by the mucopolysaccharidoses. The higher prevalence seen in the UAE is attributable to the greater proportion of consanguineous marriages. LSDs with high prevalence in this community include $G_{M1}$-gangliosidosis, MPS VII, and fucosidosis [61].

It has been suggested the birth prevalence may be higher than previously appreciated for certain conditions, such as Fabry disease; although pilot screening programs appear to include a large proportion of patients believed to have an attenuated form of the condition; i.e., characterized by later onset of symptoms, in which case newborn screening may create a dilemma regarding the appropriate time to initiate therapy, and also the issue of diagnosis in the case of minors [62].

The prevalence data and availability of disease-modifying therapies have prompted interest in the potential inclusion of certain LSDs to a panel representing a further expansion of newborn screening program (which has included screening for fatty acid oxidation disorders, following the introduction of tandem mass spectrometry).

A wide range of laboratory tests may be used for diagnosis of LSDs, but the most frequently employed assays are based on measurement of enzyme activity using artificial substrates in dried blood spot (DBS) on filter paper by tandem mass spectrometry measurement of substrates and their turnover. This approach allows a multiplex setup, adapted for high-throughput screening. [*Note*: enzyme-based assays will miss rare variants resulting from co-factor deficiency, which require molecular genetic testing for confirmation. Furthermore, enzyme pseudo-deficiency may be a confounding issue (e.g., ARSA), and assay of enzyme activity can lead to indiscriminate detection not only of classically affected, early-onset cases, but those at risk for attenuated clinical expression as well.]

It is likely, future screening or early diagnosis programs will incorporate sequencing methods involving selected candidate genes, in place of or to complement current biochemical assays. A potential issue with DNA based assays is the identification of variants of uncertain significance, primarily in a setting where there is no clearly affected relative to assess the pattern of segregation. This has been raised as a concern in general population screening programs for Fabry disease [63]. With increased therapeutic options, there may be opportunities for an individualized approach (so called '*personalized medicine*'). It has been suggested, screening assays (e.g., oxysterol levels in patients suspected to have NPC) may be incorporated into a tiered approach towards diagnosis. In the case of the latter, sensitivity and specificity will need to be established, prior to implementation.

Newborn screening for an LSD (Krabbe disease) was initiated in New York State in 2006. Other countries have followed suit, with programs in Taiwan for Pompe and Fabry disease.

Among Ashkenazi Jews (of Central and Eastern European descent), the high frequency of four LSDs (*viz.*, Gaucher, Tay-Sachs[32], Niemann-Pick type A and Mucolipidosis IV) has prompted inclusion of these conditions in extant carrier screening programs (for several diseases that are prevalent within the community) [64]. Among the Ultra-Orthodox, this program has been part of so-called 'suitable' marriage arrangements (*sidduch*).

Other screening programs have focused on detection of undiagnosed cases within defined patient groups, such as those with cardiomyopathy and/or renal failure (for Fabry disease) or Parkinsonian features (Gaucher disease), in whom testing for more common etiologies has not enabled a causal diagnosis [65]. In these instances, there is the added potential benefit for those identified as a result of cascade screening (i.e., testing of relatives, who may be presymptomatic or misdiagnosed when the proband has been diagnosed). The basis of the increased risk for Parkinson among carriers and affected individuals with Gaucher disease is the subject of intense investigations; currently, there is no means for predicting which individuals with Gaucher disease, or are a carrier of this trait, will develop this co-morbidity.

Screening programs will need to be supported by an infrastructure, maintained on the technical side by staff with the requisite apparatus, reagents and knowhow; employing techniques whose sensitivity and specificity have been evaluated. Clinical staff must be prepared to provide appropriate counselling and have expertise with assessment of disease severity, and with proficiency to aid with making decisions regarding the initiation of therapy and appropriate follow up. Access to therapy, if available and its reimbursement will also have to be worked outin advance. Although treatment

[32] Tay-Sachs disease (TSD) is an autosomal recessive LSD, caused by deficiency of the enzyme β-Hexosaminidase A (α-subunit), characterized by neurodegenerative features and the presence of a cherry red spot (an eye finding wherein the reddish macula is made prominent by the surrounding accumulation of gangliosides in retinal ganglion cells which give it a yellowish discoloration). Mutations of the β-subunit of β-Hexosaminidase A is the cause of Sandoff disease, associated with features that overlap with TSD.

may be available, as noted a significant proportion of patients continue to experience disease complications, which should be raised as a possibility so expectations are managed and patients counselled appropriately. Other issues revolve around testing of minors and counselling of presymptomatic adults at risk for attenuated phenotypes (so-called '*patient-in-waiting*'); diagnosed but not treated as of yet.

In summary, advances in the last two decades have led to significant improvement in the lives of affected individuals and their families. It is anticipated the next few years will expand the number of potentially treatable conditions. A range of options will also enable selection of the treatment most suitable to patient circumstances. Meanwhile, preventive approaches are available, and for those in whom there are no disease-specific therapies it must be appreciated that attention to associated problems, such as alterations of sleep-wake cycle, swallowing problems, seizures, etc. can led to significant improvement in quality of life. Ideally, care should be comprehensive and delivered through centers of excellence with multidisciplinary expertise.

## References


[1] Neufeld EF. Fro2011. m serendipity to therapy. *Annu Rev Biochem.* 80:1-15.

[2] Aldenhoven M, Wynn RF, Orchard PJ, O'Meara A, Veys P, Fischer A, Valayannopoulos V, Neven B, Rovelli A, Prasad VK, Tolar J, Allewelt H, Jones SA, Parini R, Renard M, Bordon V, Wulffraat NM, de Koning TJ, Shapiro EG, Kurtzberg J, Boelens JJ.2015. Long-term outcome of Hurler syndrome patients after hematopoietic cell transplantation: an international multicenter study. *Blood.* 125(13):2164-72.

[3] Duffner PK, Caviness VS Jr, Erbe RW, Patterson MC, Schultz KR, Wenger DA, Whitley C. 2009. The long-term outcomes of presymptomatic infants transplanted for Krabbe disease: report of the workshop held on July 11 and 12, 2008, Holiday Valley, New York. *Genet Med.* 11(6):450-4.

[4] Breen C, Wynn RF, O'Meara A, O'Mahony E, Rust S, Imrie J, Wraith JE. 2013. Developmental outcome post allogenic bone marrow transplant for Niemann Pick Type C2. *Mol Genet Metab.* 108(1):82-4.

[5] Watson HA, Holley RJ, Langford-Smith KJ, Wilkinson FL, van Kuppevelt TH, Wynn RF, Wraith JE, Merry CL, Bigger BW. 2014. Heparan sulfate inhibits hematopoietic stem and progenitor cell migration and engraftment in mucopolysaccharidosis I. *J Biol Chem.* 289(52):36194-203.

[6] Kuehn SC, Koehne T, Cornils K, Markmann S, Riedel C, Pestka JM, Schweizer M, Baldauf C, Yorgan TA, Krause M, Keller J, Neven M, Breyer S, Stuecker R, Muschol N, Busse B, Braulke T, Fehse B, Amling M, Schinke T. 2015. Impaired bone remodeling and its correction by combination therapy in a mouse model of mucopolysaccharidosis-I. *Hum Mol Genet.* 24(24):7075-86.

[7] Iglesias DM, El-Kares R, Taranta A, Bellomo F, Emma F, Besouw M, Levtchenko E, Toelen J, van den Heuvel L, Chu L, Zhao J, Young YK, Eliopoulos N, Goodyer P. 2012. Stem cell microvesicles transfer cystinosin to human cystinotic cells and reduce cystine accumulation *in vitro. PLoS One.* 7(8):e42840.

[8] Lee H, Lee JK, Min WK, Bae JH, He X, Schuchman EH, Bae JS, Jin HK. 2010. Bone marrow-derived mesenchymal stem cells prevent the loss of Niemann-Pick type C mouse Purkinje neurons by correcting sphingolipid metabolism and increasing sphingosine-1-phosphate. *Stem Cells.* 28(4):821-31.

[9] Ripoll CB, Flaat M, Klopf-Eiermann J, Fisher-Perkins JM, Trygg CB, Scruggs BA, McCants ML, Leonard HP, Lin AF, Zhang S, Eagle ME, Alvarez X, Li YT, Li SC, Gimble JM, Bunnell BA. 2011. Mesenchymal lineage stem cells have pronounced anti-inflammatory effects in the twitcher mouse model of Krabbe's disease. *Stem Cells.* 29(1):67-77.

[10] Scruggs BA, Zhang X, Bowles AC, Gold PA, Semon JA, Fisher-Perkins JM, Zhang S, Bonvillain RW, Myers L, Li SC, Kalueff AV, Bunnell BA. 2013. Multipotent stromal cells alleviate inflammation, neuropathology, and symptoms associated with globoid cell leukodystrophy in the twitcher mouse. *Stem Cells.* 31(8):1523-34.

[11] Coulson-Thomas VJ, Caterson B, Kao WW. 2013. Transplantation of human umbilical mesenchymal stem cells cures the corneal defects of mucopolysaccharidosis VII mice. *Stem Cells* 31(10):2116-26.

[12] Pelekanos RA, Ting MJ, Sardesai VS, Ryan JM, Lim YC, Chan JK, Fisk NM. 2014. Intracellular trafficking and endocytosis of CXCR4 in fetal mesenchymal stem/stromal cells. *BMC Cell Biol.* 15:15.

[13] Brady RO, Barton NW. 1994. Enzyme replacement therapy for Gaucher disease: critical investigations beyond demonstration of clinical efficacy. *Biochem Med Metab Biol*. 52(1):1-9.

[14] Ko Y, Lee C, Moon MH, Hong GR, Cheon CK, Lee JS. 2015. Unravelling the mechanism of action of enzyme replacement therapy in Fabry disease. *J Hum Genet*.

[15] Weidemann F, Sanchez-Niño MD, Politei J, Oliveira JP, Wanner C, Warnock DG, Ortiz A. 2013. Fibrosis: a key feature of Fabry disease with potential therapeutic implications. *Orphanet J Rare Dis*. 8:116.

[16] Patel V, O'Mahony C, Hughes D, Rahman MS, Coats C, Murphy E, Lachmann R, Mehta A, Elliott PM. 2015. Clinical and genetic predictors of major cardiac events in patients with Anderson-Fabry Disease. *Heart*. 101(12):961-6.

[17] Falk DJ, Todd AG, Lee S, Soustek MS, ElMallah MK, Fuller DD, Notterpek L, Byrne BJ. 2015. Peripheral nerve and neuromuscular junction pathology in Pompe disease. *Hum Mol Genet*. 24(3):625-36.

[18] Harmatz P. 2015. Enzyme replacement therapies and immunogenicity in Lysosomal storage diseases: Is there a pattern? *Clin Ther*.

[19] Stenger EO, Kazi Z, Lisi E, Gambello MJ, Kishnani P. 2015. Immune tolerance strategies in siblings with infantile Pompe disease-Advantages for a preemptive approach to high-sustained antibody titers. Mol Genet Metab Rep. 4:30-34.

[20] Han SO, Pope R, Li S, Kishnani PS, Steet R, Koeberl DD. 2015. A beta-blocker, propranolol, decreases the efficacy from enzyme replacement therapy in Pompe disease. *Mol Genet Metab*.

[21] Koeberl DD, Austin S, Case LE, Smith EC, Buckley AF, Young SP, Bali D, Kishnani PS. 2014. Adjunctive albuterol enhances the response to enzyme replacement therapy in late-onset Pompe disease. *FASEB J*. 28(5):2171-6.

[22] Papademetriou J, Garnacho C, Serrano D, Bhowmick T, Schuchman EH, Muro S. 2013. Comparative binding, endocytosis, and biodistribution of antibodies and antibody-coated carriers for targeted delivery of lysosomal enzymes to ICAM-1 versus transferrin receptor. *J Inherit Metab Dis*. 36(3):467-77.

[23] Hsu J, Northrup L, Bhowmick T, Muro S. 2012. Enhanced delivery of α-glucosidase for Pompe disease by ICAM-1-targeted nanocarriers: comparative performance of a strategy for three distinct lysosomal storage disorders. *Nanomedicine*. 8(5):731-9.

[24] Hsu J, Serrano D, Bhowmick T, Kumar K, Shen Y, Kuo YC, Garnacho C, Muro S. 2011. Enhanced endothelial delivery and biochemical effects of α-galactosidase by ICAM-1-targeted nanocarriers for Fabry disease. *J Control Release*.149(3):323-31.

[25] Boado RJ, Lu JZ, Hui EK, Sumbria RK, Pardridge WM. 2013. Pharmacokinetics and brain uptake in the rhesus monkey of a fusion protein of arylsulfatase a and a monoclonal antibody against the human insulin receptor. *Biotechnol Bioeng*. 110(5):1456-65.

[26] Prince WS, McCormick LM, Wendt DJ, Fitzpatrick PA, Schwartz KL, Aguilera AI, Koppaka V, Christianson TM, Vellard MC, Pavloff N, Lemontt JF, Qin M, Starr CM, Bu G, Zankel TC. 2004. Lipoprotein receptor binding, cellular uptake, and lysosomal delivery of fusions between the receptor-associated protein (RAP) and alpha-L-iduronidase or acid alpha-glucosidase. *J Biol Chem*. 279(33):35037-46.

[27] Böckenhoff A, Cramer S, Wölte P, Knieling S, Wohlenberg C, Gieselmann V, Galla HJ, Matzner U. 2014. Comparison of five peptide vectors for improved brain delivery of the lysosomal enzyme arylsulfatase *A. J Neurosci*. 34(9):3122-9.

[28] Venier RE, Igdoura SA. 2012. Miglustat as a therapeutic agent: prospects and caveats. *J Med Genet*. 49(9):591-7.

[29] Lyseng-Williamson KA. 2014. Miglustat: a review of its use in Niemann-Pick disease type C. *Drugs*. 74(1):61-74.

[30] Cox TM, Drelichman G, Cravo R, Balwani M, Burrow TA, Martins AM, Lukina E, Rosenbloom B, Ross L, Angell J, Puga AC. 2015. Eliglustat compared with imiglucerase in patients with Gaucher's disease type 1 stabilised on enzyme replacement therapy: a phase 3, randomised, open-label, non-inferiority trial. *Lancet*. 385(9985):2355-62.

[31] Mistry PK, Lukina E, Ben Turkia H, Amato D, Baris H, Dasouki M, Ghosn M, Mehta A, Packman S, Pastores G, Petakov M, Assouline S, Balwani M, Danda S, Hadjiev E, Ortega A, Shankar S, Solano MH, Ross L, Angell J, Peterschmitt MJ. 2015. Effect of oral eliglustat on splenomegaly in patients with Gaucher disease type 1: the ENGAGE randomized clinical trial. *JAMA*. 313(7):695-706.

[32] Brandvold KR, Morimoto RI. 2015. The chemical biology of molecular chaperones-implications for modulation of proteostasis. *J Mol Biol*. 427(18):2931-47.

[33] Germain DP, Giugliani R, Hughes DA, Mehta A, Nicholls K, Barisoni L, Jennette CJ, Bragat A, Castelli J, Sitaraman S, Lockhart DJ, Boudes PF. 2012. Safety and pharmacodynamic effects of a pharmacological chaperone on α-galactosidase A activity and globotriaosylceramide clearance in Fabry disease: report from two phase 2 clinical studies. *Orphanet J Rare Dis.* 7:91.

[34] Warnock DG, Bichet DG, Holida M, Goker-Alpan O, Nicholls K, Thomas M, Eyskens F, Shankar S, Adera M, Sitaraman S, Khanna R, Flanagan JJ, Wustman BA, Barth J, Barlow C, Valenzano KJ, Lockhart DJ, Boudes P, Johnson FK. 2015. Oral Migalastat HCl leads to greater systemic exposure and tissue levels of active α-Galactosidase A in Fabry patients when co-administered with infused Agalsidase. *PLoS One.* 10(8):e0134341.

[35] Bartolomeo R, Polishchuk EV, Volpi N, Polishchuk RS, Auricchio A. 2013. Pharmacological read-through of nonsense ARSB mutations as a potential therapeutic approach for mucopolysaccharidosis VI. *J Inherit Metab Dis.* 36(2):363-71.

[36] Gunn G, Dai Y, Du M, Belakhov V, Kandasamy J, Schoeb TR, Baasov T, Bedwell DM, Keeling KM. 2014. Long-term nonsense suppression therapy moderates MPS I-H disease progression. *Mol Genet Metab.* 111(3):374-81.

[37] Miller JN, Kovács AD, Pearce DA. 2015. The novel Cln1(R151X) mouse model of infantile neuronal ceroid lipofuscinosis (INCL) for testing nonsense suppression therapy. *Hum Mol Genet.* 24(1):185-96.

[38] Tanaka Y, Yamada Y, Ishitsuka Y, Matsuo M, Shiraishi K, Wada K, Uchio Y, Kondo Y, Takeo T, Nakagata N, Higashi T, Motoyama K, Arima H, Mochinaga S, Higaki K, Ohno K, Irie T. 2015. Efficacy of 2-Hydroxypropyl-β-cyclodextrin_in Niemann-Pick Disease Type C Model Mice and Its Pharmacokinetic Analysis in a Patient with the Disease. *Biol Pharm Bull.* 38(6):844-51.

[39] Song W, Wang F, Lotfi P, Sardiello M, Segatori L. 2014. 2-Hydroxypropyl-β-cyclodextrin promotes transcription factor EB-mediated activation of autophagy: implications for therapy. *J Biol Chem.* 289(14):10211-22.

[40] Matsuo M, Togawa M, Hirabaru K, Mochinaga S, Narita A, Adachi M, Egashira M, Irie T, Ohno K. 2013. Effects of cyclodextrin in two patients with Niemann-Pick Type C disease. *Mol Genet Metab.* 108(1):76-81.

[41] Maarup TJ, Chen AH, Porter FD, Farhat NY, Ory DS, Sidhu R, Jiang X, Dickson PI. 2015. Intrathecal 2-hydroxypropyl-beta-cyclodextrin_in a single patient with Niemann-Pick C1. *Mol Genet Metab.*

[42] Moskot M, Montefusco S, Jakóbkiewicz-Banecka J, Mozolewski P, Węgrzyn A, Di Bernardo D, Węgrzyn G, Medina DL, Ballabio A, Gabig-Cimińska M. 2014. The phytoestrogen genistein modulates lysosomal metabolism and transcription factor EB (TFEB) activation. *J Biol Chem.* 289(24):17054-69.

[43] Warnock DG, Thomas CP, Vujkovac B, Campbell RC, Charrow J, Laney DA, Jackson LL, Wilcox WR, Wanner C. 2015. Antiproteinuric therapy and Fabry nephropathy: factors associated with preserved kidney function during agalsidase-beta therapy. *J Med Genet.* 52(12):860-6.

[44] Boentert M, Karabul N, Wenninger S, Stubbe-Dräger B, Mengel E, Schoser B, Young P. 2015. Sleep-related symptoms and sleep-disordered breathing in adult Pompe disease. *Eur J Neurol.* 22(2):369-76.

[45] Kishnani PS, Steiner RD, Bali D, Berger K, Byrne BJ, Case LE, Crowley JF, Downs S, Howell RR, Kravitz RM, Mackey J, Marsden D, Martins AM, Millington DS, Nicolino M, O'Grady G, Patterson MC, Rapoport DM, Slonim A, Spencer CT, Tifft CJ, Watson MS. 2006. Pompe disease diagnosis and management guideline. *Genet Med.* 8(5):267-88.

[46] Slonim AE, Bulone L, Goldberg T, Minikes J, Slonim E, Galanko J, Martiniuk F. 2007. Modification of the natural history of adult-onset acid maltase deficiency by nutrition and exercise therapy. Muscle Nerve. 35(1):70-7.

[47] Seehafer SS, Ramirez-Montealegre D, Wong AM, Chan CH, Castaneda J, Horak M, Ahmadi SM, Lim MJ, Cooper JD, Pearce DA. 2011. Immunosuppression alters disease severity in juvenile Batten disease mice. *J Neuroimmunol.* 230(1-2):169-72.

[48] Williams IM, Wallom KL, Smith DA, Al Eisa N, Smith C, Platt FM. 2014. Improved neuroprotection using miglustat, curcumin and ibuprofen as a triple combination therapy in Niemann-Pick disease type C1 mice. *Neurobiol Dis.* 67:9-17.

[49] Narita K, Choudhury A, Dobrenis K, Sharma DK, Holicky EL, Marks DL, Walkley SU, Pagano RE. 2005. Protein transduction of Rab9 in Niemann-Pick C cells reduces cholesterol storage. *FASEB J.* 19(11):1558-60.

[50] Helquist P, Maxfield FR, Wiech NL, Wiest O. 2013. Treatment of Niemann--pick type C disease by histone deacetylase inhibitors. *Neurotherapeutics.* 10(4):688-97.

[51] Macías-Vidal J, Girós M, Guerrero M, Gascón P, Serratosa J, Bachs O, Coll MJ. 2014. The proteasome inhibitor bortezomib reduced cholesterol accumulation in fibroblasts from Niemann-Pick type C patients carrying missense mutations. *FEBS J.* 281(19):4450-66.

[52] Barranger JA, Rice EO, Dunigan J, Sansieri C, Takiyama N, Beeler M, Lancia J, Lucot S, Scheirer-Fochler S, Mohney T, Swaney W, Bahnson A, Ball E. 1997. Gaucher's disease: studies of gene transfer to haematopoietic cells. *Baillieres Clin Haematol.* 10(4):765-78.

[53] Kotterman MA, Chalberg TW, Schaffer DV. 2015. Viral vectors for gene therapy: Translational and clinical outlook. *Annu Rev Biomed Eng.* 17:63-89.

[54] Biffi A, Montini E, Lorioli L, Cesani M, Fumagalli F, Plati T, Baldoli C, Martino S, Calabria A, Canale S, Benedicenti F, Vallanti G, Biasco L, Leo S, Kabbara N, Zanetti G, Rizzo WB, Mehta NA, Cicalese MP, Casiraghi M, Boelens JJ, Del Carro U, Dow DJ, Schmidt M, Assanelli A, Neduva V, Di Serio C, Stupka E, Gardner J, von Kalle C, Bordignon C, Ciceri F, Rovelli A, Roncarolo MG, Aiuti A, Sessa M, Naldini L. 2013. Lentiviral hematopoietic stem cell gene therapy benefits metachromatic leukodystrophy. *Science.* 341(6148):1233158.

[55] Zerah M, Piguet F, Colle MA, Raoul S, Deschamps JY, Deniaud J, Gautier B, Toulgoat F, Bieche I, Laurendeau I, Sondhi D, Souweidane MM, Cartier-Lacave N, Moullier P, Crystal RG, Roujeau T, Sevin C, Aubourg P. 2015. Intracerebral Gene Therapy Using AAVrh.10-hARSA Recombinant Vector to Treat Patients with Early-Onset Forms of Metachromatic Leukodystrophy: Preclinical Feasibility and Safety Assessments in Nonhuman Primates. *Hum Gene Ther Clin Dev.* 26(2):113-24.

[56] Tardieu M, Zérah M, Husson B, de Bournonville S, Deiva K, Adamsbaum C, Vincent F, Hocquemiller M, Broissand C, Furlan V, Ballabio A, Fraldi A, Crystal RG, Baugnon T, Roujeau T, Heard JM, Danos O. 2014. Intracerebral administration of adeno-associated viral vector serotype rh.10 carrying human SGSH and SUMF1 cDNAs in children with mucopolysaccharidosis type IIIA disease: results of a phase I/II trial. *Hum Gene Ther.* 25(6):506-16.

[57] Ruzo A, Garcia M, Ribera A, Villacampa P, Haurigot V, Marcó S, Ayuso E, Anguela XM, Roca C, Agudo J, Ramos D, Ruberte J, Bosch F. 2012. Liver production of sulfamidase reverses peripheral and ameliorates CNS pathology in mucopolysaccharidosis IIIA mice. *Mol Ther.* 20(2):254-66.

[58] Yin H, Kanasty RL, Eltoukhy AA, Vegas AJ, Dorkin JR, Anderson DG. 2014. Non-viral vectors for gene-based therapy. *Nat Rev Genet.* 15(8):541-55.

[59] Quiviger M, Arfi A, Mansard D, Delacotte L, Pastor M, Scherman D, Marie C. 2014. High and prolonged sulfamidase secretion by the liver of MPS-IIIA mice following hydrodynamic tail vein delivery of antibiotic-free pFAR4 plasmid vector. *Gene Ther.* 21(12):1001-7.

[60] Yin H, Xue W, Chen S, Bogorad RL, Benedetti E, Grompe M, Koteliansky V, Sharp PA, Jacks T, Anderson DG. 2014. Genome editing with Cas9 in adult mice corrects a disease mutation and phenotype. *Nat Biotechnol.* 32(6):551-3.

[61] Al-Jasmi FA, Tawfig N, Berniah A, Ali BR, Taleb M, Hertecant JL, Bastaki F, Souid AK. 2013. Prevalence and Novel Mutations of Lysosomal Storage Disorders in United Arab Emirates: LSD in UAE. *JIMD Rep*. 10:1-9.

[62] Kingma SD, Bodamer OA, Wijburg FA. 2015. Epidemiology and diagnosis of lysosomal storage disorders; challenges of screening. *Best Pract Res Clin Endocrinol Metab*. 29(2):145-57.

[63] Linthorst GE, Bouwman MG, Wijburg FA, Aerts JM, Poorthuis BJ, Hollak CE. 2010. Screening for Fabry disease in high-risk populations: a systematic review. *J Med Genet*. 47(4):217-22.

[64] Hoffman JD, Park JJ, Schreiber-Agus N, Kornreich R, Tanner AK, Keiles S, Friedman KJ, Heim RA. 2014. The Ashkenazi Jewish carrier screening panel: evolution, status quo, and disparities. *Prenat Diagn.* 34(12):1161-7.

[65] Lesage S, Anheim M, Condroyer C, Pollak P, Durif F, Dupuits C, Viallet F, Lohmann E, Corvol JC, Honoré A, Rivaud S, Vidailhet M, Dürr A, Brice A; French Parkinson's Disease Genetics Study Group. 2011. Large-scale screening of the Gaucher's disease-related glucocerebrosidase gene in Europeans with Parkinson's disease. *Hum Mol Genet*. 20(1):202-10.

# About the Author

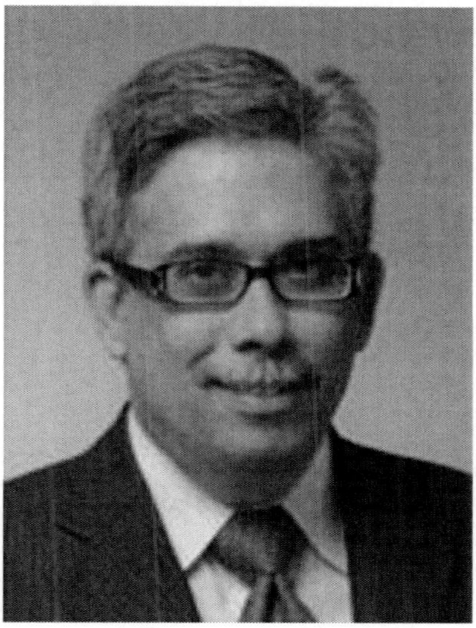

**Gregory M. Pastores, MD,** is a Consultant with the Adult Metabolic Service/Department of Medicine/National Centre for Inherited Metabolic Disorders at the Mater Misericordiae University Hospital, Eccles Street, Dublin 7, Ireland.

Dr. Pastores is also an Associate Clinical Professor, University College Dublin, Ireland, and Visiting Professor with the Department of Medicine, Yale University School of Medicine, New Haven, CT, USA.

A graduate of the University of Sto. Tomas in Manila (1983), he trained in Pediatrics and Genetics at the Mount Sinai Medical Center in New York

(1989) and at the Mayo Clinic in Minnesota (1991). While at Mount Sinai, he received the Young Pediatric Investigator Award, Mount Sinai Child Health Research Center, NIH (5 P30 HD28822), 1993-1996, and the Clinical Associate Physician Award, Mount Sinai General Clinical Research Center, National Center for Research Resources, NIH (5M01-RR0071), 1996-1997.

Prior to coming to Ireland, he was an Associate Professor of Neurology and Pediatrics at the NYU School of Medicine in New York, and Director of the Neurogenetics Laboratory for the Department of Neurology at NYU (1997-2013).

Dr. Pastores has Board Certification in Pediatrics (1989), Clinical Genetics (1993) and Clinical Molecular Genetics (1993). He has extensive clinical and research experience in the diagnosis and management of patients with the lysosomal storage disorders, and was engaged in the development and testing of treatments for Gaucher, Fabry, MPS I, IVa and VI, Pompe disease and a late (adult)-onset form of Tay-Sachs disease ($G_{M2}$-gangliosidosis). He has published over 250 papers, 25 book chapters and two textbooks.

# Index

## C



## D

## E



## F



## G



## H

## I



## K



## L



## M

## N



## O



## P

## Q



## R



## S